Navigating in a Crisis: Lessons for Mexico in the COVID-19 Context

NAVIGATING IN A CRISIS

LESSONS FOR MEXICO IN THE COVID-19 CONTEXT

DANIEL TAPIA QUINTANA

EDITOR

Westphalia Press
An Imprint of the Policy Studies Organization
Washington, DC
2021

August 2021

NAVIGATING IN A CRISIS: LESSONS FOR MEXICO IN THE COVID-19 CONTEXT

GC Genera

Public policy consulting firm specialized in the analysis, design, implementation, and evaluation of public policies. We focus on the development of evidence-informed policy decisions to improve project performance and drive positive change and optimal outcomes for our clients on the public, private and social sectors.

GC · G · E · N · E · R · A

Puebla, Mexico

10 AÑOS

www.gcgenera.com

Published by Westphalia Press
An imprint of Policy Studies Organization
1527 New Hampshire Ave., NW
Washington, D.C. 20036
www.ipsonet.org

ISBN: 978-1-63723-603-1

PSO

Policy Studies Organization
Washington, DC

Contents

Acknowledgments

This book was conceived throughout the development of COVID-19 in Mexico and focused on the analysis of the multiple effects and implications derived from this pandemic. In GC Genera's effort to generate added value, we consider that this phenomenon, initially of public health, should be approached from additional areas of public interest with a more pragmatic and purposeful vision.

In April 2020, we began reviewing studies, international and national editorials, and academic reports about the pandemic, its repercussions, and strategies implemented by the authorities. Moreover, we participated in webinars and analyzed documents and considered all relevant information at the international and national level about the COVID-19 pandemic. In this way, this project took shape, intending to underline a series of reflections about the consequences and develop recommendations to address the pandemic.

First, I would like to acknowledge the invaluable contribution of each one of my colleagues who participated in the development of this book.

This effort would not have been possible without the collaboration of Cecilia García Montoya, Carol Daniela Aceval Carmona, Marcela Reynoso Jurado, Maribel Flores Sánchez, Rosángel Hernández Mendoza, Esteban Santamaría Hernández, José Carlos Espinoza Lanz, Juan Carlos Baker Pineda, and Pedro Manuel Lichtle Fragoso. I deeply appreciate your commitment for sharing, from your areas of expertise and experience, the implications of the pandemic and its effects in different areas such as citizenship, commerce, political communication, creative economy, education, penitentiary system, tourism, and gender violence.

I would also like to thank the support of Hugo Cimadevilla, Joel Aranda Ávila, and Jonathan Torres Trejo, who, with their contributions, strengthened the development of this project. This book would not have been possible without their talent and dedicated effort.

Daniel Tapia Quintana
Executive Director
GC Genera

Introduction

After more than 15 months of the emergency caused by the COVID-19 pandemic, health authorities reported more than 197 million cases and more than 4.2 million deaths globally. In Mexico, at the beginning of August 2021, there were more than 2.8 million people infected and around 240,000 deaths.

At the international level, we are experiencing unprecedented health, social, and economic crises in constant evolution as evidenced by new variants of the virus presented in the United Kingdom, South Africa, and Italy, among others. When the vaccines' distribution begins to generate hope internationally, new mutations threaten countries in their quest to stop the illness through stricter lockdowns.

In the first quarter of 2020, many countries stopped essential and non-essential activities resulting in significant, mostly negative, impacts on the population. Specifically, in Latin America, complex social problems such as poverty, inequality, and marginalization increased in a context of popular discontent, public mistrust, and growing tensions between society and authorities.

As the pandemic evolved, these problems worsened. The crisis's impact will have devastating consequences in health, education, and employment, affecting all population groups: children, youth, adults, and the elderly. This crisis has shown that the problems are not exclusive to certain groups or social sectors; on the contrary, they represent a public matter whose solution concerns everyone involved.

Several countries have had to face the pandemic with diverse capacities and resources. COVID-19 has become a severe test for global leadership and, specifically, health, education, finance, and labor systems. The pandemic has exposed one of the evident problems in many Latin American countries, especially Mexico: we spend badly, inefficiently, and opaquely, which results in unequal and poor-quality education, health, and safety systems. Day by day, we witnessed a greater number of shreds of evidence that demonstrate the deficit of personnel, Intensive Care Units (ICU), and medical equipment as hospitals struggle to treat all people with symptoms of COVID-19 throughout the Mexican territory.

In a context where different countries of the world face severe or flexible lockdowns and with the reopening of economic and commercial activities, the recovery will depend on the measures adopted by governments to stimulate the economy, promote actions to support the most vulnerable population, and close the gaps that the pandemic will leave in health, employment, and education, just to mention a few.

Likewise, the success or failure of containing the COVID-19 virus will lie in the capacity of public actors, private, and social organizations in coordinating actions to reduce the scale, magnitude, and spread of the disease through public policies and programs that benefit a greater number of people.

Under the direction of GC Genera, the book was developed with experts' support with extensive experience in eight areas where Mexico will face challenges in the context of the COVID-19 pandemic: citizenship, commerce, political communication, creative economy, education, penitentiary system, tourism, and gender violence.

At the time of publishing this book, we know that the pandemic is not over. For that reason, we consider it of utmost importance to analyze how and under what conditions we are dealing with the disease and identify how we can address this challenge to prevent further human losses and, therefore, political, social, and economic instability in our country.

We want this book to be a tool for crisis management and prevention of problems derived from externalities that may affect the future prospects of the country at the national, state, and local levels. We hope it may serve as a lesson to compensate for past mistakes and to rethink solutions based on evidence to avoid further human losses and other economic effects.

Finally, we hope that policymakers and people involved in analyzing, designing, and implementing public policies in Mexico find this book useful as we intend it to become an invitation to reflect, debate, and develop better public policies for the solution of public affairs.

The Path Towards the Transformation of Tourism in Mexico: Lessons from COVID-19

Pedro Lichtle

Tourism in Mexico, like many other sectors, is suffering from a profound crisis as a consequence of the pandemic caused by COVID-19 and the global economy's deceleration. However, as one of the gross domestic product's (GDP) major components and one of the main sources of foreign exchange income in Mexico, its downturn impacted the country's development and, specifically, local economies that depend on this activity to a greater extent.

Expectations for global tourism's recovery, under current conditions, focus on regional and local tourism dynamics. It has been speculated that travelers will avoid overcrowded tourist spots, will make shorter trips, and will seek sanitary safety in their destinations. Mexico must undertake a greater commitment to this. Although the Ministry of Tourism (Secretaría de Turismo or SECTUR) has established safety measures for reactivation and prioritized domestic tourism as a key element in the sector's recovery, it is paradoxical that before the pandemic, policies to boost this sector had been undermined.

Bearing this approach in mind, the purpose of this analysis is to recommend strategies that will allow decision-makers and public policy designers to carry out precise actions to invigorate the tourism industry. Such strategies are aimed towards strengthening tourist offer at destinations and encouraging the domestic market's demand. They do not attempt to solve the complex situation of national and global tourism activity, but they do seek to serve as a guide when designing solutions that will ease the sector's negative impact.

Tourism's Relevance Before COVID-19

Towards the second half of 2019, international tourism was regarded with great encouragement by the World Tourism Organization (WTO). The international tourist arrivals index increased by 5% with 1,400 million arrivals, and tourist exportation increased by 4%, reaching 1.7 trillion dollars. The industry represented 3.6% of the world GDP. Zurab Pololikashvili, the WTO's Secretary-General, then stated that the strength shown made the industry a true global driving force for growth and development (WTO, 2019).

In 2018, Mexico occupied the 7th place world-wide in international tourist arrivals, with more than 41.5 million arrivals, ranking above global powers such as Germany and the United Kingdom. Tourism represented 8.7% of the GDP and created 6% of the country's gainful occupations. It earned a place as one of the main sources of foreign exchange, along with remittances and oil, according to the 2019 Mexico Tourism Satellite Account published by the Instituto Nacional de Estadística y Geografía (National Insitute of Statistics and Geography, INEGI).

In contrast, its economic revenue was smaller. The diagnosis provided by the Estrategia Nacional de Turismo (National Tourism Strategy) 2019-2024 suggested that, in 2018, Mexico had ranked 16th in tourist expenditure and 40th in expenditure per tourist.

Outside Mexico City, 84.7% of international tourism congregated around five tourist destinations. Domestic tourism was the strongest component in the country's tourism activity, as approximately 8 out of every 10 Mexican pesos spent on tourism came from domestic consumption.

Consequently, the strategy suggested strengthening the southeastern region, dividing destinations by region, increasing expenditure per international tourist, producing livelihood for inhabitants of tourist destinations, and diversifying the attractions market. However, the suggested action plan and budget assigned did not respond to aspirations for the sector.

On the one hand, the goal was to breach the gap in the development of national tourism and to boost domestic tourism. However, 3 out of the 5 strategies focused on the international market: market diversification, international tourism expenditure increase, and southeastern tourism consolidation. In order to achieve this last strategy, Mexico's government is building a railroad (Tren Maya) in the Yucatan Peninsula, whose main pull factor will be international tourism.

On the other hand, national tourism's institutional capabilities were weakened through budget cuts and the disappearance of institutions. In 2020, the Presupuesto de Egresos de la Federación (Federal Budget or PEF) showed a decline of more than 40% in SECTUR resources in comparison to 2019, specifically, in the budget allocated to projects that promote domestic tourism such as Pueblos Mágicos (Magical Towns Programme), a Mexican tourism policy with wide world recognition. Additionally, the Consejo de Promoción Turística de México (Mexican Council for Tourism Promotion or CPTM) was canceled and its advertising role was delegated to the Ministry of Foreign Affairs, with limited knowledge and resources.

Before the pandemic, the Mexican government reduced the sector's institutional capabilities and public policy actions were not linked to the suggested strategy, at least regarding domestic tourism. This would harm local tourism policy, which to a certain extent, depended on budgetary programs destined for regional tourist development and advertising.

The Tourism Sector in the Face of the Pandemic

The first case of the disease caused by COVID-19 was announced on December 31st, 2019, in Wuhan, China. Weeks later, as the virus expanded, the World Health Organization (WHO) sent out a statement on January 27th, 2020, suggesting measures that would limit the risk of transmission during international travel without, yet restricting it. The disease's rapid spread led WHO to declare a pandemic on March 11th, 2020.

The WTO spoke out in favor of health without restricting travel by initially asking travelers to conduct tourism responsibly in the face of the current situation. Nevertheless, several countries and regions started to implement more restrictive measures, such as the closing of borders or the cancellation of international flights. For example, the European Union announced the closing of borders on March 17th, and the United States announced its tourism restrictions on March 20th. Global tourism's dynamics collapsed rapidly. The WHO declared on April 28th that 100% of destinations worldwide had implemented traveling restrictions.

The health crisis quickly started to reflect on the sector's economic perspectives. According to the International Tourism Barometer in May (WTO, 2020), between 60 and 80% of international tourism was expected to drop during 2020 and 120 million direct jobs would be lost. Only within the first trimester, when travel restrictions were not abundant, international tourism shrank by 22%. International tourism's outlook was radically different from that of a few months prior.

COVID-19 arrived subsequently to Mexico. The federal government announced the "Jornada de Sana Distancia" on March 24th, 2020. Some states, businesses, and universities had started lockdown a few days before. Although this was not mandatory, it limited several tourism activities, such as accommodation services, food and drink services, performances, conferences, etc. Additionally, the mobility of the population was restricted as a consequence of transportation restrictions and other local measures like the closing of state borders or even the closing of destinations by communities themselves.

In July, INEGI reported that in Mexico, during the first quarter of 2020, international tourist arrival dropped by 24.4% in comparison to 2019's first quarter. As evidence of the crisis' severity, international tourist arrival decreased by 78.5% in April compared to the same month in 2019. Nonetheless, border tourism's loss was less dramatic; it reduced by 13.2% during the first quarter, suggesting that, despite the closing of borders, the frontier's dynamics avoided a greater decline for tourism in Mexico. This was probably due to specific dynamics in these areas. Remittances' revenue figures warned of a further decrease by dropping 34% during 2020's first quarter. Not only did fewer tourists arrive, but their expenses were also less. Such reduction shows a change in tourists' behavior patterns.

Hotel activity dropped as well, according to DATATUR's website (a tourism open data platform). On the one hand, 2020's first-quarter hotel occupancy, which refers to the number of rooms taken in relation to the current total offer, was 34.1% below 2019's. By April, the situation was even more dramatic as it decreased by 94.8%. On the other hand, the number of occupied rooms diminished by 32%. It is important to point out that this number does not consider total room availability but allows the identification of tourists' origins. Rooms occupied because of domestic tourism decreased by 34.1%, which represented five percentage points greater than international tourists'.

Furthermore, the number of tourists per night in hotels also shrank by 32.1%, making the drop in national tourists' figure, 34.6%, greater than that of international ones by six percentage points. This index reflects tourists' stay in hotel rooms, that is, the number of nights they spend at the establishment.

These data suggested that not only had traveler arrival decreased, but that hotel room demand had fallen at a greater scale. Additionally, it was possible to observe that, often, fewer rooms were required for domestic tourism than for international tourism, suggesting, then, the size of tourist groups reduced, trips were shorter, and Mexican travelers were more receptive to confinement measures or traded hotel rooms for other types of accommodation services, such as staying at relatives' homes.

This shows that although the international tourism reduction caused by COVID-19 impacted Mexico in the arrival ofboth domestic and international tourism, changes in the behavior of demand in both sectors occurred at different scales.

The New Normal and the Sector's Recovery

The new normal implied the return to activities carried out routinely before the pandemic, taking into consideration that, without a vaccine against COVID-19, the disease would persist. This situation brought up a dilemma. On the one hand, the best measure to control the spread of the virus was the population's confinement. On the other hand, people needed to leave their homes to reactivate economic sectors.

By the end of August 2020, the spread of COVID-19 had surpassed thirty million cases and almost one million deaths worldwide. Geographically, the situation was different. While in some regions the virus' spread had decreased, this had not yet occurred in others. Sadly, the American continent was in the spotlight, particularly the United States, where 30% of the world's contagion and one-fourth of global deaths had been registered. At the moment of the analysis' conclusion, figures beyond 684,000 cases and 72,000 deaths have been registered in Mexico.

Given this situation, there was no certainty about the moment in which COVID-19 cases would be controlled or tourist destinations would re-open. However, some of the dangers included making rushed decisions, increasing risks for tourists and communities, and dividing tourism in Mexico as a consequence of such diverse recovery actions.

Economic prospects also showed a complex panorama. There was a negative consensus regarding 2020's end of the year expectations. The World Bank predicted that the global economy would shrink by 5.2%, the International Monetary Fund (IMF) foretold a 4.9% drop, Fitch Ratings estimated it at 4.6%, and Morgan Stanley at 3.8%, among others. In the United States' case, Mexico's main source of tourists, the economic outlook was also weak. A 6.1% fall and an unemployment rate of 20% were expected for the United States' economy in 2020. However, the dollar had appreciated about 16% in relation to the Mexican currency during the first semester of the year. Yet Americans' trips to Mexico were expected to continue declining. According to Sanchez and Cruz (2016), fluctuations in American travelers' incomes explained almost 40% of their traveling intentions, and dollar appreciation another 13%.

The country's economy was also fragile. The World Bank's estimate for Mexico considered a drop of 7.5% for 2020, the Economic Commission for Latin America and the Caribbean (ECLAC) calculated it at 9%, and BBVA estimated it at 10% or 11.2%, according to Citibanamex.

In June, INEGI reported that, according to their consumer confidence survey published in May, more than 30% of the economically active population (EAP) was unemployed or underemployed and that only 16.8% of consumers perceive the economic possibilities of going on vacation during the following twelve months.

In this light, in June 2020, the WTO foresaw behavior changes in travelers, who would seek sustainable tourism, thus, focusing on the importance of domestic tourism for the industry's recovery.

In order to re-open and re-activate tourism activity in Mexico, it was necessary to restore tourists' trust, to give them certainty about their sanitary safety, and to understand tourists' new behavior patterns while considering global and regional economic perspectives.

By then, some initiatives to increase tourists' confidence had already developed in Mexico. Through the Federal Government, SECTUR announced the guidelines to resume several tourism activities in the national territory in May 2020. This, in collaboration with different business chambers, associations, interest groups, and the main tourist-destination-states in the country. Additionally, it spread a few promotional videos on social media aimed at attracting international tourists. It also held meetings with the private sector to develop a digital marketing strategy through the Visit Mexico search engine. However, none of these strategies contained actions to directly support businesses or tourism employment.

Separately, local governments implemented diverse measures to re-open and re-activate their economic activities. Firstly, different reopening dynamics created confusion. For example, the state of Sinaloa had announced the reopening of the hotel sector on June 8th, but then delayed it. The state of Veracruz announced hotel reopening from June 15th on with a maximum occupancy of 25% of their capacity. The state of Guanajuato authorized hotel reopening at a maximum occupancy of 30% from June 8th on.

Secondly, public policy proposals for recovery lacked coherence and coordination, risking their effectiveness during their implementation. For example, the state of Quintana Roo proposed a Tourist Sanitary Certification for businesses, while the state of Chiapas chose to return hotel occupancy taxes and payroll taxes to tourism companies as well as 50% of total state toll prices to tourists within the state's territory. Although the differences in strategies responded to each state's characteristics and market, they also produced uncertainty and wariness due to the lack of coordination and standardization. This situation risked dividing tourism destinations.

Finally, tourism companies also implemented their own strategies. Some hotel chains declared obtaining certifications for tourist safety and the facility sanitization. These endeavors were essential to recover tourist confidence and to reduce traveler uncertainty but were insufficient if they were not adopted by the entire travel offer. For example, a hotel certification was not useful for travelers if safety measures in transportation, gas services, drug stores, department stores, or malls were not standardized.

In conclusion, both travelers and businesses will continue facing risks and uncertainty due to the new normal's health, economic and tourism prospects. This would produce higher costs according to Vitoriano's (2007) decision-making models, which, in turn, would reflect on prices paid by tourists, according to Williams and Baláž (2015). The lack of coordination among the different parts of the tourism industry and the misalignment of policies within the country would imply a cost increase for tourists. This would play against the goal of reactivating internal demand.

Suggestions to Transform Tourism in Mexico

The tourism industry showed resilience to the 2008 financial crisis and after AH1N1 influenza. However, COVID-19's context is different. National tourism policies' institutional weakness, the health crisis' characteristics, and economic expectations for the near future lay out a unique scenario. The tourism industry's recovery will not happen spontaneously. It is necessary to reduce risk and uncertainty as well as to inspire confidence in tourists.

This experience teaches a lesson for tourism in Mexico: it is necessary to have public policies and tools to promote domestic tourism, as well as mechanisms to foster policy transversality for the sector. Additionally, this has drawn attention to the importance of ensuring the industry's resilience, taking advantage of internal demand, and enhancing tourism's institutional capacity. Consequently, three policy suggestions aimed at transforming the Mexican tourism industry are laid out below.

1.Management and Regularization of Tourist Offerings

The first suggestion is to manage and standardize tourist supply. The main goal is to gain a full understanding of tourism activities in the national territory to develop better tourism strategies to enhance the supply and safety of the demand, as well as to react appropriately and effectively when facing any sort of risk.

The management programs should include the following characteristics: Geography of natural resources, geography of risks, economic activities, infrastructure, urban morphology, as well as population flow and density.

With this outlook on management, it will be possible to access geographical and statistical information that will allow the creation of better civil protection and planning for municipalities. Considering the current sanitary context, this would require a better knowledge of tourism spaces, of the maximum guest density allowed in establishments and popular tourism areas, of the population groups interacting with tourists, among others. This would lead to structuring more precise containment strategies in the face of possible disease outbreaks without shutting down activities completely, and would help crime prevention, tourist traceability, and the economy.

The regularization of tourist offer is aimed at ensuring all establishments in tourist destinations abide by local regulations. This by seeing that they have operating licenses, sanitary and public safety measures that guarantee the establishment's proper functioning, and tourist protection. A well-implemented strategy would avoid excessive regulations that may result in discouraging innovation and entrepreneurship. Nonetheless, the business sector should become aware that regulating does not mean controlling, but rather strengthening the industry.

Underlying the idea of regularization is the possibility of ensuring that tourism industry meets the minimum requirements for operating. This, in turn, will bring the government certainty about compliance with regulations and the elements to take on the responsibility tourists need regarding the quality and care in tourist destinations and services.

Additionally, within the Mexican federalist framework, the tax effort of municipalities may benefit given the payment of licenses that local regulations imply, since, according to Guzman et al. (2015), on average, municipalities with tourism activity collect more and depend less on federal contribution than the national average. These resources could then be used to strengthen the municipalities' development and tourist development.

Finally, management and regularization will offer a wider array of elements for governance. If management is understood and implemented in line with the General Tourism Law (Ley General del Turismo) and its regulations, as well as the regularization of tourist establishments is carried out in a moderate manner, they will allow for a greater capacity and coordination that will enhance institutional capabilities among different governmental spheres and parties involved in tourism activities (Rosas, 2008).

Both land-use planning in municipalities of a touristic nature and the regularization of tourist industry within a municipality's territory represent opportunities for tourism activity. The current situation legitimizes and lays out the precise moment to develop both activities.

2. Development of Regional Tourism

The second strategy is to develop regional tourism. This refers to tourism trips that take place in a specific region of similar geographical or cultural traits. The proposal revolves around the development of regional strategies that challenge geographical municipal or state borders.

In Mexico, like in many other parts of the world, the nature of tourist destinations and political geography is intertwined. Hence, local governments tend to see the tourism industry through the perspective of local promotion rather than as a form of productive linkage. This produces competing public policies in sometimes neighboring destinations. This approach aims to establish coordinating and mutual consent policies between municipalities and states to complement tourism supply thus attracting more tourists, increasing the length of overnight stays, increasing economic revenue, and managing destinations sustainably.

Currently, global phenomena have altered travelers' behavior in this sense. Sustainable and regional tourism has become increasingly coveted. Tourism activity has outlined landscapes that extend beyond political borders. Collective efforts for tourism policies with a regional approach will allow reducing uncertainty and risks for travelers while standardizing measures in regional tourist destinations, services, and products.

The government must align action frameworks and working schemes. Cooperation between authorities and parties involved in the regional tourism will enable making the necessary adjustments in a timely and effective manner. Within this perspective, it would be possible to manage destinations more efficiently, for example, when directing visitor flow and density among all tourist attractions in the region.

For instance, if a tourist attraction has reached the maximum guest density allowed according to social distancing standards required by the new health regulations or by guidelines in wilderness areas, activity coordination and concurrence between states and municipalities could promote information exchange to distribute visitors across the region. This would adequately fulfill their needs without damaging nature, the infrastructure, or the facility's image.

Lastly, based on Cervantes and Gomez's (2007) suggestions, regional tourism strategies could mend current imbalances, considering the tourist phenomenon in a given territory is an intricate system due to the existing relations between the host society, tourists, transit pathways, productive activity, and natural, sanitary, economic, social and political hazards.

Developing regional tourism, then, will allow strengthening tourist offer, addressing changes in touristic demand, increasing economic revenue, enhancing destinations' sustainability, and mending current imbalances while improving coordination between the federation, states, and municipalities.

3. *An Inclusive Digital Transformation of Tourist Offerings*

The third strategy is to digitally transform tourist offerings in an inclusive manner. Digital transformation refers to a change process undergone to improve tourism operations through the use of digital technology. This idea does not only rely on the use of technology, but on organizational change, structure, leadership, and the team in charge of the change process as well. These aspects are often more important than technological ones.

In the face of global dynamics, investing in the digital transformation of all tourism services, products, and destinations in Mexico is a necessity and a way of protecting tourism businesses in the face of global dynamics. An example of this would be strengthening the domestic market. Sanitary restrictions drew attention to the need for e-commerce, diversified domestic demand, and fostered the re-distribution of local and regional markets. For example, the new dynamic imposed by lockdown restrictions led to the need for delivery or take-out services. Graph 1 shows search tendencies for the terms "delivery services," "take-out," and "stay home" between February 15th and May 31st, 2020 on the Google Search Engine. States with the highest number of searches for "delivery services" were Nuevo Leon, Yucatan, Colima, Quintana Roo, Sinaloa, Baja California, Jalisco, Aguascalientes, and Tabasco. It is possible to observe that the situation sparked other needs, causing a new structure for domestic market and market diversification.

In the absence of tourists, in municipalities with tourism activity, several businesses and services were able to take advantage of demand or to offer alternatives that placed them under the eye of a new captive market by providing delivery or take-out services. Not all businesses were able to react in the same way, as there was a lack of digital mediums (such as mobile apps to locate services, stores, or customized assistance) to do so. To exemplify this proposal, having a directory containing all tourist services in a single mobile app for the destination could boost economic activities during confinement. In addition to this, making tourist transportation digital could incentivize their use for delivery or shipping services. Making businesses digital could also help to quantify density in tourist destinations, manage guest flow, and improve destination's tourist traceability, among others, the analysis of information and the implementation of technologies such as artificial intelligence.

Graph 1. *Google Searches in Mexico (February 15th to May 31st, 2020).*

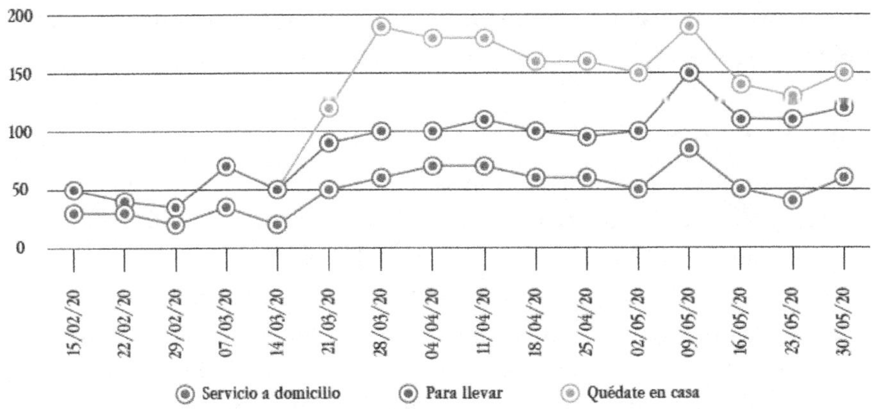

Source: Prepared by the author based on Google Trends data, 2020.

Consequently, tourism businesses and governments must opt to promote innovation culture, leadership focused on change and the development of technology skills among the most important strategies. The goal is to take advantage of technological and innovation opportunities to develop businesses that allow, on one hand, providing resilience in the face of crisis and, on the other hand, adapting more quickly and efficiently to situations.

Lastly, these three suggestions are important for the transformation of the tourism sector in Mexico. However, it is necessary to continue identifying more trends regarding new demands' behavior. This would allow the planning of new public policies, designing new schemes for promotion and commercialization, as well as the transformation of the industry according to tourism's new standards.

The previously described proposals can be implemented individually but executing all three will produce a greater positive impact. Strong knowledge about the destination, along with clear planning, will doubtlessly contribute to the coordination and management of tourist offerings. Having regional strategies will make tourism more attractive, promote sustainability, and encourage market diversification. Finally, technology's assistance will take advantage of conditions established by travelers and destinations to produce a greater economic revenue that will benefit the community's development. It is important to recognize that national tourism policies force local governments and other parties in the tourism industry to collaborate, even more so in the new global setting. In light of this, solutions must be creative and precise.

Final Thoughts

Economic activity in Mexico, especially in some states and municipalities is deeply dependent on tourism. Mobility restrictions, confinement and wariness caused by COVID-19 were factors that showed the sector's fragility. Traveler absence limited economic conditions for the development of many regions and populations. While depending on a single economic activity is a problem in itself, it is impossible to deny the country's reality, which proves that tourism represents an opportunity for development, and given the lack of opportunities, it is sometimes the only one.

The health crisis and its economic impact brought up the need to change and improve Mexican tourism strategies. Covid-19's arrival and development provided lessons about the advantages and disadvantages of tourism activity. Currently, it is necessary to favor sustainable tourism, protect domestic tourism, and promote the industry's resilience. To achieve this, it would be necessary to regulate tourist offer, adopt regional tourism dynamics, and undertake digital transformation of the industry.

COVID-19 is a turning point in global dynamics. However, it should be the starting point for the transformation of tourism activity in Mexico. Thus, a new ideal for tourism will be promoted; it will not merely be a source of income for Mexico, but also a part of environmental protection, supporting its workers and their families, promoting internal demand, and creating development in Mexico.

Bibliography

Banco Mundial. (2020). *Global Economic Prospects*. Washington, D.C.: Banco Mundial.

Carbajal de Nova, C., and Goicoechea, J. (2014). Consumo privado por origen y componente: efectos ingreso y precio para México. Investigación Económica, 73(289). Retrieved from: http://www.scielo.org.mx/scielo.php?script=sci_arttext&pid=S0185-16672014000300005

Cervantes, J., and Gómez, R. (2007). El ordenamiento territorial como eje de planeación de proyectos de turismo sustentable. *Ciencias Sociales 4* (2), 103 118.

Diario Oficial de la Federación. (2015). Reglamento de la Ley General de Turismo. Retrieved from: http://www.diputados.gob.mx/LeyesBiblio/regley/Reg_LGT_160817.pdf

Diario Oficial de la Federación. (2019). Presupuesto de Egresos de la Fed-eración para el ejercicio fiscal 2019. México. Retrieved from: http://www.diputados.gob.mx/sedia/biblio/prog_leg/Prog_leg_LXIV/010_DOF_28dic18.pdf

Diario Oficial de la Federación. (2020). Presupuesto de Egresos de la Federación para el ejercicio fiscal 2020. México. Retrieved from: http://www.diputados.gob.mx/LeyesBiblio/ref/pef_2020.htm

Fondo Nacional de Fomento al Turismo. (s.f.). Tren Maya, Análisis costo beneficio, versión pública. Retrieved from: https://www.trenmaya.go b.mx/

Guzmán, M. et al. (2015). Esfuerzo Fiscal Municipal en Destinos Turísticos. SECTUR. Documentos de Investigación Estadística y Económica, 2015-04. Retrieved from: http://www.datatur.sectur.gob.mx/Documentos%20Publicaciones/2015_4_DocInvs.pdf

Instituto Nacional de Estadística y Geografía. (2019). Cuenta Satélite del Turismo de México, 2018. (Comunicado de prensa núm. 700/19). Retrievedfrom: https://www.inegi.org.mx/contenidos/saladeprensa/boletines/2019/StmaCntaNal/CST2018.pdf

Instituto Nacional de Estadística y Geografía. (2020a). Encuestas de Viajeros Internacionales, cifras preliminares durante abril 2020. Retrieved from: https://inegi.org.mx/contenidos/saladeprensa/notasinformati vas/2020/ViajInternales/ViajInternales2020_06.pdf

Instituto Nacional de Estadística y Geografía. (2020b). Resultados de la Encuesta Telefónica sobre Confianza del Consumidor (ETCO). Retrieved from: https://www.inegi.org.mx/contenidos/saladeprensa/boletines/2020/especiales/ETCO2020_05.pdf

Instituto Nacional de Estadística y Geografía. (2020c). Resultados de la Encuesta Telefónica de Ocupación y Empleo (ETOE), cifras oportunas de abril de 2020. Retrieved from: https://www.inegi.org.mx/conteni dos/investigacion/etoe/doc/etoe_nota_tecnica_junio_2020.pdf

Organización Mundial del Turismo. (2019). *Panorama del turismo internacional*. Madrid: OMT.

Organización Mundial del Turismo. (2020a). La sostenibilidad es la nueva normalidad: una visión de futuro para el turismo. Retrieved from: https://www.unwto.org/es/covid-19-oneplanet-recuperacion-re sponsable

Organización Mundial del Turismo. (2020b). World Tourism Barometer. Retrieved from: https://www.e-unwto.org/

Rosas, A. (2008). Una ruta metodológica para evaluar la capacidad institucional. Retrieved from: http://www.scielo.org.mx/scielo.php?script=sci_ar

ttext&pid=S0188-77422008000200006

Sánchez, F. and Cruz, J. (2016). Determinantes económicos de los flujos de viajeros a México. *Revista de Análisis Económico*, 31(2), 1-19.

Secretaría de Turismo. (2019). Estrategia Nacional de Turismo 2019-2024 tendrá un sentido democrático. Retrieved from: https://www.gob.mx/sectur/prensa/estrategia-nacional-de-turismo-2019-2024-tendra-un-sentido-democratico-miguel-torruco

Secretaría de Turismo. (2020). Secretarías de Salud y de Turismo presentan Lineamiento Nacional para la Reapertura del Sector Turístico. Retrieved from: https://coronavirus.gob.mx/2020/05/20/secretarias-de-salud-y-de-turismo-presentan-lineamiento-nacional-para-la-reapertura-del-sector-turistico/

Secretaría de Turismo. (2020a). Resultados de la Actividad Turística, marzo 2020. Retrieved from: https://www.datatur.sectur.gob.mx

Vitoriano, B. (2007). Teoría de la Decisión: Decisión con Incertidumbre, Decisión Multicriterio y Teoría de Juegos. Retrieved from: https://www.mat.ucm.es/~bvitoria/Archivos/a_dt_UCM.pdf

Williams, A., and Baláž, V. (2015). Tourism, risk and uncertainty: theoretical reflections. *Journal of Travel Research*, 54 (3), 271-287.

Public Policy and the Pandemic: A Threat or an Opportunity for Women's Equality?

Marcela Reynoso

Introduction

Equality is a human right recognized as universal to all human beings and it is inalienable to their human condition. From a formal approach, this concept involves acknowledging its status in regulations and procedures (Barnard & Hepple, 2000). Thus, it is stated in the constitutions and general norms that compose a society's legal framework. However, formal equality does not necessarily ensure people's access to an environment that guarantees equal conditions, and in which people can fully develop on a day-to-day basis. Even with the existence of laws and regulations, access to opportunities differs from one person to another.

From a philosophical standpoint, equality is thought of as a qualitative and relational affair. Hence, its relevance depends on the comparison of characteristics between subjects (Gosepath, 2011). In this respect, feminist theories have made a great effort to review the meaning of equality between men and women in each context, and above all, its meaning in relation to men, considering the elimination of asymmetries and domination as their main purpose (Mansbridge & Okin, 2017).

Mexico has made important advances towards formal equality. Equality is recognized by the 4th Article of the Mexican Constitution and there is also a General Law for the Equality of Men and Women (Ley General para la Igualdad de Mujeres y Hombres). On an international level, Mexico is part of the Convention on the Elimination of All Forms of Discrimination against Women (CEDAW), The Beijing Protocole, The Inter-American Convention to Prevent, Sanction and Eradicate Violence against Women (Belem do Pará), to name a few examples.

However, inequality persists in our society, placing women at a disadvantage in different spheres of life, hindering their overall development.

Public policies present alternatives to solve public dilemmas; however, it is necessary to have a holistic perspective of the realities of people whose needs differ. For this reason, intersectionality plays a vital part in the confrontation of challenges that individuals face depending on the context they find themselves in. This concept has been fundamental in generating a gender perspective that incorporates the life experiences of women and demystifying patriarchal stereotypes surrounding femininity that perpetuate gender inequality (Bubeck, 2000).

This way, gender perspective has provided a viable alternative for dealing with the lack of formal equality that has been established by regulations but is still yet to be applied. Therefore, formulating the concept of "Substantive equality" requires a tool that can distinguish the access to truly equal conditions. This is why its existence on paper contributes to the removal of gender gaps. However, as it was previously pointed out, equality has been conceived in relation to male-dominated contexts in society, and public policies that intend to guarantee access to such, presume that the environments in which men and women develop are equal. The COVID-19 pandemic has not been an exception to this.

The Position of Women in Mexico: Where Were We, Before the Pandemic?

Before the outbreak of the COVID-19 crisis, gender disparity was already reflected in the conditions that drove Mexican women to the edge and that enabled the fitting protests that took place during March 2020 (Reynoso & Schietekat, 2020). The social demands made by Mexican women reflected the depth of the gaps and the lack of opportunities that they face and that affect the overall development of women in the country.

An aggravating issue that permeates the life of women is the violence against them. In Mexico, two out of three (66.1%) of the 46.5 million women over the age of 15 have reported experiencing some form of violence in their life. And 53.2% of the times, the perpetrator is their romantic partner (INEGI, 2018). This is quite a sensitive and worrying issue, as it represents a threat to the integrity of women that can yield irreversible consequences such as death.

It is estimated that 10 women die in Mexico every day, victims of femicide (Velázquez, 2019). Even though this is considered a criminal offense, there are fundamental flaws in the execution of the factors that contribute to this process. Estimates indicate that, when it comes to crimes committed against women, only 6.3% of them are investigated (INEGI,2019). As can be seen, while these crimes are well regulated through general laws and criminal codes, the reality eludes justice. Women remain the victims of a violence that they seem unable to escape and cannot rely on the support of public policies to solve the issue.

Women are also at a disadvantage when it comes to work-related issues. On the one hand, according to a study conducted by the National Council for the Prevention of Discrimination (CONAPRED), the wage gap in Mexico is estimated to be 34.2% per work hour (Solis, 2017), which represents devaluation of women's work and inhibits their professional growth. On the other hand, women spend significantly more time on household activities than men. Women put in 76% of their time towards domestic housework and home care, men put 23.6%. This is also unpaid labor (INEGI, 2019).

Health wise, maternal deaths were already delicate matter. In 2019, the ratio was 30 deaths per 100 thousand births. The Organization for Economic Co-operation and Development (OECD) average is 18 deaths. There were relevant factors that contributed to these numbers in addition to the direct and indirect causes, such as lack of medications and distance to healthcare centers, among others (García Martínez, 2020).

Additionally, an important element for the analysis surrounding women in the country is education. In Mexico, women experience the biggest educational gap, considering gender and age, older women suffer a bigger disadvantage (INEA, 2015). This means that the lack of the necessary knowledge ostracizes women from taking part in important areas of their daily life, such as: personal finances, contract signing, using electronic devices like computers or apps that facilitate their activities, inserting themselves in a more competitive labor market, finishing more complex tasks in a shorter period, staying up to date or avoid losing their job as a result of automation.

The digital gap is another important factor for the analysis of the structural disadvantages faced by women in Mexico. Nonetheless, there are no indicators created specifically to measure this, that is, without even taking gender perspective into consideration. The educational gap indicators serve as a proxy, as they measure gaps in necessary knowledge of basic technology use left by primary and secondary education. However, the problem still lacks visibility, as a result of the absence of statistics.

As shown, the scenarios faced by Mexican women are complex and involve unequal access to opportunities and overall development. The following section reviews how the previously discussed unequal conditions have exacerbated by the public policies put into place in an effort to mitigate the issues related to the pandemic. These policies still lack gender perspective.

The Position of Women in the COVID-19 Pandemic

After a brief diagnosis of the issues that affect the lives of women in Mexico, it is possible to contrast it to what developed during the handling of the COVID-19. It is necessary to provide context on how the Mexican authorities handled the pandemic, and how it affected women. This is an illustrative but not restrictive contextualization of the initiatives held to handle the pandemic.

Domestic Violence

When the pandemic began, the predominant measure taken was confinement. Regarding this, the government held an information campaign called "Quédate en casa"[1] or "Stay at Home," which promoted voluntary self-isolation to lower the risk of contagion due to activities held outside. This campaign was developed due to an official release on March 27, 2020 by the Ministry of Health (Secretaría de Salud), in which they "mandate immediate suspension from March 30 to April 30, 2020, of all non-essential activities, in order to mitigate the spread of SARS-CoV2 in the community..." (DOF, 2020). In light of the situation presented by home isolation, it is important to consider that under normal circumstances, some women are already assaulted by their romantic partners. Confinement, predictably served as the triggering factor to perpetrate more violence against women.

And, as expected, violence has increased: The National Shelter Network, estimated that between March and June 2020, the number of women, girls, and boys under the care of an association increased 81% in comparison to the same period in 2019 (Animal Político, 2020). According to the same organization, the kinds of violence that have been reported the most are physical assault (41.15%), emotional violence (23.29%), economic and property violence (5.46%), and sexual violence (3.63%) (RNR, 2020).

To deal with this situation, the federal government introduced the "Count to Ten" campaign, as a strategy to fight violence against women during the pandemic. The campaign manifested itself in the form of videos and images telling people to "remain calm" and "do not despair." This campaign ignores that domestic violence happens in three-stage cycles: tension, crisis, and regret, and that remaining calm is not enough to avoid violence. Additionally, the video fails to address the previously mentioned fact that the violence suffered by women is mainly perpetrated by their romantic partners. Quite the contrary, it discusses violence in personal relationships and therefore should not be used as an instrument to assist women.

Furthermore, the Federal Government's Coronavirus website has a section dedicated to gender violence. This section lists the measures taken to deal with this issue during the pandemic. Unfortunately, the site lacks gender perspective, and it does not have specific actions aimed at addressing the surge in the rate of violence. Rather, they establish general measures based on gender stereotypes that characterize women as weak and helpless.

On the other hand, the support line provided for women in violent situations does not specialize in violence against women, as it would require gender perspective to be employed. The "Lifeline" (800 911 2000) is geared towards the general public and specializes in addiction and mental health (CONADIC, 2018). Meanwhile, line 800 HÁBLALO (Speak it) was, unfortunately, disconnected. The line provided free legal and psychological counseling with gender perspective for women who suffered violence. It was open 24 hours a day, 365 days a year, and sought the well-being of women through personalized follow- ups for each case (Gob.mx, 2016). It is important to point out that violence is a crime that requires specialized care, especially, after such an increase of violence, like the one seen during the pandemic.

To deal with this issue and avoid a setback in the fight to eradicate violence against women, specific measures must be implemented. There have been good international practices on that matter: for example, Spain established a service to provide psychological council through WhatsApp and carried out an awareness campaign. The Czech Republic trained delivery employees to recognize signs of violence, and Slovenia conducted an intensive program that works with offenders via Zoom.

Implementing specific public policy measures means acknowledging the pressing matters: First, the existence and severity of the situation. Second, recognizing that it must be dealt with in a pointed matter to safeguard the integrity of women. In Mexico, unfortunately, this has yet to be addressed.

Forms of Work (Formal and Informal)

Lock-down as a basic measure to prevent the spread has also had a severe impact economically, not just in Mexico, but in several countries worldwide. According to Alicia Bárcena, Executive Secretary for the Economic Commission for Latin America and the Caribbean (CEPAL), in Mexico, 500 thousand formal businesses will close due to the pandemic (Meza, 2020).

Likewise, it is estimated that 11.6 million people have lost their jobs, most of them being women and young people (Xatomila, 2020). Additionally, a relevant fact is that 55% of the people working in the service industry are women (Durant, 2020). This suggests that they will be most affected by the impacts of the pandemic, which have mainly harmed this industry (UNCTAD, 2020).

On the other hand, in terms of unpaid work, it is important to point out that women provide most of the caregiving in the country's current scenario. On top of this, given the suspension of work activities, it is estimated that the amount of housework has tripled for women since the start of the pandemic (Reynoso & Schietekat, 2020).

Education

In terms of education, the halt in work activities due to the lock-down may lead to a halt in the education of women in the country. As previously discussed, violence against women and girls has increased in their homes during the pandemic. This may translate in an increase of unplanned pregnancies, or pregnancies as a result of sexual violence, an overload of housework, and an increase in physical and psychological violence. These factors could inhibit the development of women and their educational achievements, or even, bring about the end of their studies. Educational authorities in Mexico need to provide effective solutions so that this pandemic does not further hinder education and widen the educational gap for women.

This situation is alarming, as it adds to the preexisting educational gap which makes it impossible for women to occupy jobs in the scientific field. According to UNESCO (2019), only 29.3% of jobs in the scientific field are occupied by women. This may be related to gender roles and stereotypes that are yet to be dispelled. The current circumstances caused by the pandemic, force women to copy these behavioral models and might represent a setback in this aspect.

Digital Gap

The digital gap is intrinsically tied to education. Regarding the use of technology, it is important to discuss that the migration to digital media due to the need for long-distance communication, may significantly affect women.

According to the Inter-American Development Bank (BID): Mexico has a significant gender-gap in terms of internet access: 49% of men, compared to 38% of women (BID, 2020).

Furthermore, 40% of Latin-American women do not know how to use the internet, and without the proper necessary policies, as technology advances women will remain unable to use it. Conversely, this situation can also be tied to work related issues. According to a report written by the British Embassy (2018), the manufacture and construction industries rely heavily on technology and are predominantly male dominated. Based on this study, estimates suggest that automation (using machines or apps to perform tasks previously done by humans), would take over 19% of the jobs in these industries. Therefore, greater skills in the use of Artificial Intelligence (AI) would be necessary to mitigate job loss.

This shift will probably be greater due to the heavy use of AI, in which women are not very involved. In this sense, action is necessary to avoid widening the gap between men and women when it comes to technological knowledge. Thus, preventing women from missing out on jobs that require such skills is a priority.

Both local and national governments need to identify the biggest gaps and setbacks that women already face in relation to men. These gaps may be exacerbated after the pandemic due to the normalized use of new technologies.

Physical and Mental Health

Regarding maternal death, the "Guidelines for the Prevention and Mitigation of COVID-19 during Pregnancy Care, Delivery, Postpartum and Newborns," were published in April to prevent and mitigate an increase in maternal deaths associated with the pandemic. However, COVID-19 became the leading cause of maternal death after the 28th epidemiological week with 17.8% of deaths confirmed (Secretaría de Salud, 2020). After the 30th epidemiological week the number had increased to 18.5%; a ratio of 39.8 deaths per 100 thousand confirmed births. This is estimated to be 21.2% higher in comparison to the same epidemiological week of 2019 (Secretaría de Salud, 2020).

According to Dr. Hilda Argüello Avedaño, Technical Secretary of the Maternal Mortality Observatory of Mexico, scientific evidence shows that the virus doesn't necessarily increase the deaths of women during pregnancy, labor or postpartum. Indicating a possible cause could be the lack of protocols and guidelines to prevent the spread (García Martínez, 2020). Furthermore, the increase could be attributed to causes such as the shutdown of medical facilities that previously provided timely care for complications during gestation.

The lack of hospital treatment contributes to obstetric violence. It does not just affect women during pregnancy, labor and postpartum; it also has an impact in routine subjects. These subjects include counseling regarding sexual and reproductive health, birth control and pregnancy termination, as well as the access to menstrual products and other general gynecology topics. This reaffirms the urgency to characterize obstetric violence as a type of violence against women. Furthermore, according to the National Population Council (CONAPO) and the United Nations Fund for Population Activities (UNFPA), it is expected that the surge in obstetric and sexual violence, will result in about 171,000 unplanned pregnancies, 35,000 more than the expected trend.

Lastly, due to the increase in violence against women, job loss, the large amount of unpaid work, designing public policies must be imperative to diminish these problems. These policies should look after the mental health of women, especially considering the overwhelming conditions they face (Reynoso & Schietekat, 2020).

Recommendations

There are still plenty of challenges to overcome regarding gender disparity in Mexico. On top of this, the COVID-19 pandemic and the public policy measures taken up until this point, may worsen the gaps. Thus, setting back the advances that had been made towards achieving a substantial equality that will reflect on the life of women when compared to men.

In this sense, there is an urgent need to implement measures to avoid further setbacks and disparities. The following measures are suggested as a way to achieve a more comprehensive public policy, avoiding ulterior economic and human right costs that confinement may have for women.

Immediate Actions:

- Gender perspective must be implemented across all public policies regarding the pandemic.

As discussed in the text, this would require a situational analysis of the gaps the pandemic has created on the diverse areas of women's lives. This text highlighted at least five: domestic violence, work-related (paid and unpaid), education, the digital gap, and physical and mental health. However, this list is not conclusive and there are other areas in which the disparities could increase.

- Internationally, there are some good measures to combat violence as a result of lock- down. These measures could be adapted to Mexican context.

The previously mentioned experiences of Spain and the Czech Republic using social networks such as WhatsApp and food delivery services may be a useful way to provide support for women in violent settings. Additionally, these measures do not require a budget and can be implemented at a local level.

Medium-term Actions:

- Have the necessary indicators in place to measure the rates of violence and other issues that affect the lives of women.

Suitable indicators are imperative to understand the dynamics that women find themselves in. Sex-disaggregation is not sufficient for prospective public policy planning. To do this, it is necessary to know the relevant issues that women face and to compile information from local and state entities. In this way, public policy will be able to efficiently handle emerging situations and prevent further incidence.

- Implementing measures that will involve educating men on gender disparity.

Lastly, from the standpoint of improving emotional management, deconstructing masculinity, and respecting women's rights; men should be involved in discussions regarding gender issues. It is extremely important for men to assimilate measures that implement gender perspective. These measures will allow for a more equal society and will deal with issues tied to dignity and respect towards women as human beings. Furthermore, it is important for men to understand disparities, as they are sometimes difficult to perceive since they are normalized, minimized, and even socially invisible.

Final Thoughts

As previously discussed, gender-related drivers of inequality already existed before COVID-19. These drivers have been exacerbated by the pressing situation regarding the pandemic and its handling. Relying on public policies that implement gender perspective is fundamental in correctly addressing the issues that target women and put them at a disadvantage in relation to men. This includes the previously mentioned: violence against women, paid and unpaid work, the educational and digital gaps, as well as physical and mental health. Governments have to take special care to implement specific measures that can provide adequate solutions and avoid perpetuating stereotypes and gender disparity.

Additionally, there have been policies regarding women in the past. These policies do not address the need to prepare men for the integration of women into spaces that have traditionally been unwelcoming or banned for women. This, not only applies to physical spaces, but also to positions of power. It is critical for society as a whole to accept that women have the right to occupy public spaces, to have jobs, to raise their voice and to denounce injustice, to feel free in their own bodies, and to say "no" without facing physical or social backlash.

Finally, a key message that this situation has left us is, even though this pandemic has widened the gaps of disparity, it has also given us the opportunity to realize the need for complementary public policy and new indicators with gender perspective. Government authorities in charge of providing solutions to public problems at all levels must respond to this situation with the adequate measures. Beyond the pandemic, this threatens the equality of women with regards to men and we must consider it as an opportunity to correct the path of public policy.

Bibliography

Animal Político. (2020). Violencia contra mujeres e hijos aumenta 81% durante pandemia, alertan refugios. Retrieved from: https://www.animalpolitico.com/2020/07/violencia-mujeres-hijos-aumenta-pandemia-refugios/

Barnard, C., and Hepple, B. (2000). Substantive Equality. *The Cambridge Law Journal*, Vol. 59, No. 3, 564.

Banco Interamericano de Desarrollo. (2020). Brechas digitales de género en tiempos de COVID-19. Disponible en: https://blogs.iadb.org/igualdad/es/brechas-digitales-de-generocovid-19/

British Embassy. (2018). Rumbo a una estrategia de Inteligencia Artificial. Retrieved from: https://www.gobiernohabil.com/2018/09/rumbo-una-estrategia-de-inteligencia.html

Bubeck, D. (2000). Feminism in political philosophy. Women's difference. En J. Hornsby, M. Fricke, & J. H. Fricke (Ed.), *The Cambridge companion to feminism in philosophy*. Cambridge: University Press.

Comisión Nacional contra las Adicciones. (2018). Centro de atención ciudadana La Línea de la Vida. Retrieved from: https://www.gob.mx/salud/conadic/acciones-y-programas/centro-de-atencion-ciudadana-contra-las-adicciones-134381

Diario Oficial de la Federación. (2020). ACUERDO por el que se establecen acciones extraordinarias para atender la emergencia sanitaria generada por el virus SARS-CoV2. Retrieved from: https://www.dof.gob.mx/nota_detalle.php?codigo=5590914&fecha=31/03/2020

Durant, I. (2020). COVID-19 requires gender-equal responses to save economies. Retrieved from: https://unctad.org/en/pages/newsdetails.aspx?OriginalVersionID=2319

European Commission. (2020). The EU Mutual Learning Programme in Gender Equality. Retrieved from: https://ec.europa.eu/info/sites/info/files/aid_development_cooperation_fundamental_rights/mlp_webinar_on_domestic_violence_and_covid-19_summary_report_may_2020_en.pdf

Forbes. (2019). México tiene la peor brecha salarial de género de Latinoamérica: informe. Retrieved from: https://www.forbes.com.mx/mexico-tiene-la-peor-brecha-salarial-entre-hombres-y-mujeres-informe/

García Martínez, A. (2020). México, único país de América Latina donde la muerte materna se incrementó por COVID. Retrieved from: https://cimacnoticias.com.mx/2020/07/20/mexico-unico-paisde-al-donde-la-muerte-materna-se-incremento-por-covid

Gobierno de México. (2016). ¡Si sufres violencia no estás sola! 01– 800 Háblalo. Retrieved from: https://www.gob.mx/gobmx/articulos/si-sufres-violencia-no-estas-sola-01-800-hablalo

Gobierno de México. (2020). Violencia de género. Retrieved from: https://coronavirus.gob.mx/violencia-de-genero/

Gosepath, S. (2011). Equality. Retrieved from: https://plato.stanford.edu/archives/spr2011/entries/equality/

Instituto Nacional para la Educación de los Adultos. (2015). Población de 15 años o más en rezago educativo. Retrieved from https://www.gob.mx/cms/uploads/attachment/file/174218/rez_ei15_gen_edad_hi_nal.pdf

Instituto Nacional de Estadística y Geografía. (2016). Encuesta Nacional sobre la Dinámica de las Relaciones en los Hogares. Retrieved from: https://www.inegi.org.mx/programas/endireh/2016

Instituto Nacional de Estadística y Geografía. (2018). Estadísticas a propósito del día internacional para erradicar la violencia contra las mujeres. Retrieved from: https://www.inegi.org.mx/contenidos/saladeprensa/aproposito/2018/violencia2018_Nal.pdf

Instituto Nacional de Estadística y Geografía. (2019). Cuenta satélite del trabajo no remunerado de los hogares de México. Retrieved from: https://www.inegi.org.mx/contenidos/saladeprensa/boletines/2019/StmaCntaNal/CSTNRH2019.pdf

Instituto Nacional de Estadística y Geografía. (2019). ENVIPE. Retrieved from: https://www.inegi.org.mx/programas/envipe/2019/

Mansbridge, J., and Okin, S. M. (2017). Feminism. En R. E. Goodin, P. Pettit, Thomas Pogge, R. E. Goodin, P. Pettit, & Thomas Pogge (Eds.), *A companion to contemporary political philosophy*. Blackwell.

Reynoso, M., and Schietekat, P. (2020). COVID-19, una pandemia que exacerba las desigualdades contra las mujeres. Retrieved from: http://mexicosocial.org/covid19-exacerba-desigualdades-contramujeres/

Red Nacional de Refugios. (2020). Cuatro meses de confinamiento por COVID-19 y las violencias contra las mujeres, niñas y niños continúan en aumento. Retrieved from: https://drive.google.com/file/d/1bQLKiH8jxhs-TyLONc0-GbuwR8Yg_qzCG/view

Secretaría de Salud. (2020). Informe semanal de notificación inmediata de muerte materna. Retrieved from: https://www.gob.mx/salud/documentos/informes-semanales-para-la-vigilancia-epidemiologica-de-muertes-maternas-2020

Secretaría de Salud. (2020a). Lineamiento para la prevención y mitigación de COVID-19 en la atención del embarazo, parto, puerperio y de la persona recién nacida. Retrieved from: https://www.gob.mx/cms/uploads/attachment/file/546239/Lineamiento_prevencion_y_mitigacion_de_COVID-19_en_el_embarazo_CNEGSR__1_.pdf

Solis, P. (2017). Discriminación estructural y desigualdad social. Retrieved from: https://www.conapred.org.mx/documentos_cedoc/Discriminacionestructural%20accs.pdf

United Nations Conference on Trade and Development. (2020). Coronavirus deals severe blow to services sectors. Retrieved from: https://unctad.org/en/pages/newsdetails.aspx?OriginalVersionID=2327

Velázquez, M. (2019). En promedio, 10 mujeres son asesinadas al día. Retrieved from: https://www.eleconomista.com.mx/politica/En promedio-10-mujeres-son-asesinadas-al-dia-20190409-0010.html

World Bank. (2017). Maternal mortality ratio. Retrieved from: https://data.worldbank.org/indicator/sh.sta.mmrt?most_recent_value_desc=true

Xantomila, J. (2020). Se dispara tasa de desempleo en México en 2o.

trimestre, reportan. Retrieved from: https://www.jornada.com.mx/ultimas/economia/2020/07/16/en-el-2deg-trimestre-13-millones-800-mil-perdieron-su-empleo-en-mexico-1348.html

The "New Mexican School" Model: Challenges Regarding Educational Disparity in the Context of the Covid-19 Pandemic

José Carlos Espinoza

Daniel Tapia

Throughout the last few decades, Mexico has been incapable of designing and adopting a state policy regarding education that can provide continuity and achieve the goals set out to ensure students reach an optimal learning level that allows them to develop their abilities and skills. Unfortunately, decision-makers try to re-design educational policies every six years (Sexenio is the popular term for the term limit on the President of Mexico) without providing any continuity to what has worked.

The New Mexican School (Nueva Escuela Mexicana or NEM), the new educational model implemented during the administration of President Andres Manuel Lopez Obrador, faces a major challenge. The COVID-19 pandemic has disrupted the educational reality and the foundations set for education in Mexico. If NEM initially was laid out to be an instrument of the State aiming to attain equity and educational excellence through its comprehensive improvement and maximal learning achievements, with the current situation, this premise will be difficult to accomplish.

It is important to highlight that the COVID-19 pandemic is not the source of the prevailing inequalities in the Mexican education system. That is, this public health phenomenon arrived to further amplify an already complex problem in Mexican schools. Undoubtedly, the pandemic will negatively impact the educational gap among students at a national scale for the next few years, which will imply putting in additional resources and efforts to reduce these inequalities.

All signs point to the fact that it will be complex to carry out actions and/or educational programs to guarantee the right to education from preschool to higher education for the most vulnerable and marginalized sectors—mainly those in the south and southeastern part of the country. This is also especially true among indigenous communities, afro-descendants, migrants, women, and people with disabilities. This task's complexity is the result of the social and economic effects passed on to Mexican households due to the pandemic.

It is not new for each administration to try to set itself apart from its predecessors and to try to erase its actions—regardless of whether these are good or bad—thus starting a completely new process. Nevertheless, the environment faced by the current administration as a consequence of the pandemic has been one of the main triggers of an impasse in NEM's implementation in the Mexican education system.

The COVID-19 pandemic has altered educational planning completely and interrupted already established actions and policies, radically shifting the model in a context of uncertainty. By mid-March 2020, more than 35 million students and 2 million teachers migrated from their classrooms to synchronous and asynchronous online classes, posing unthinkable challenges in terms of coverage, quality, equity, and financing.

The costs stemming from the pandemic regarding education are and will be substantial. In Mexico, a little less than half of the students received a satisfactory learning level; therefore, the current situation would further amplify this problem. According to the United Nations Development Program (2020), approximately 1.4 children and adolescents are currently at risk of permanently abandoning school. Moreover, educational gaps could be significant. According to an analysis done by Hoyos (2020), missing 60 days of learning could result in a 24-point decrease in an individual's results in a standardized test (for example, ENLACE currently known as PLANEA); hence, further postponing returning to classrooms could severely affect the future of children and youth in Mexico.

Undoubtedly, no education system worldwide was prepared to face a crisis of these proportions. However, authorities had the responsibility of responding rapidly and efficiently to the situation through the implementation of policies and measures that will mitigate the economic and educational costs of the pandemic in people's households and among the most vulnerable population. In light of the new reality, the Mexican government designed distance learning plans via the internet and television and at the same time demonstrated decision-makers' limited willingness to develop a supportive strategy or compensatory policies that would aid Mexican families that need it the most and would avoid entering a more pronounced vicious cycle of poverty and inequality.

In this way, this paper is aimed to analyze, the context of educational disparity to subsequently focus on access to Information and Communications Technologies (ITC) as an enabler to face and address the crisis. Finally, we will point out some public policy recommendations that could be useful to education decision-makers.

Educational Disparity: A Pending Task

Educational disparity is one of the greatest challenges in Mexico's educational policy (Martínez, 1992; Bracho, 1995; Székely, 1995; Muñoz Izquierdo, 1996; Schmelkes, 1997; Blanco, 2011; Esquivel, 2015; Giorguli, Vargas, Salinas, Hubert y Potter, 2015).

Mexico is formed by a vast and complex territory where there are several notable differences between each of the states. In 2018, Mexico had a GINI coefficient, an index measuring and comparing income inequality, of 0.469, one of the highest among the Organization for Economic Co-operation and Development's (OECD) member countries. As explained by Latapí (2002), substantial inequalities prevail in Mexico as a consequence of the limited access to opportunities for thousands of people, which results in an uncertain future: We are one of the countries with the greatest inequalities in the world and, additionally, we have a profoundly inequitable education system; opportunities—to access, remain and extend years of schooling, and especially to high quality and effective learning—are unequally distributed among the rich and the poor.

This extreme inequality can be observed at all educational levels when the differences in population, stratum (social and economic), area (rural-urban), or territory are compared. To summarize, the reality of education reflects social and economic inequality in our country. Educational problems such as school dropouts, access, terminal efficiency, learning, and grade failure are correlated to the aforementioned factors.

Silvia Schmelkes, a renowned professional in education, emphasizes that the path to access educational trajectory is not equal in Mexico. Inequality arises during early years and becomes perpetual through time due to socioeconomic conditions of Mexican households. To cite a particular case:

in the lowest income quintile, 55% of young people between 15 and 17 attend school; this contrasts with the 83% that attend among the highest quintile. Inequality is inherited and is one of the reasons impeding schools from becoming an apparatus that produces equality and boosts social mobility in Mexico. Finally, in Mexico, 96% of young people between the ages of 15 and 17 whose head of the family completed higher education attend school, which contrasts with 56% whose parents have no education.

The "Inequalities in Mexico" (2018) report elaborated by El Colegio de Mexico (COLMEX) highlighted that, in relation to educational performance among 15-year-old adolescents who had reached PISA level three (basic proficiency), young people with higher income have between 400 to 500% higher probability of obtaining basic proficiency in comparison to those with a lower income. On their part, women have a 20% higher probability than men of obtaining basic language proficiency, while men have a 35% higher probability of obtaining basic mathematics proficiency than women. Meanwhile, young people that do not speak an indigenous language have a 600 to 700% better probability of obtaining basic proficiency than those who speak one. Lastly, a student from an urban area has between a 300 and 400% higher chance of reaching level three than those inhabiting a rural area.

In sum, measures such as lockdown, social confinement and distancing have impacted the education system, but at different scales among students depending on their social and economic status.

Education and Technology: More Inequality or Greater Equality?

We are currently facing unprecedented conditions: the loss of a schooling space that allows interacting and socializing among different parties in the education system. In a very short period of time, systems, institutions, and educational parties had to migrate to, in some cases, an unplanned online education. The majority of countries in the world have opted for virtual education as an alternative for the progression of academic cycles. Mexico has not been an exception.

COVID-19 has accelerated the introduction of Information and Communication Technology (ICT) and digital media to the teaching and learning process at different academic levels. The education systems, specifically in Latin America, were not prepared for such change, and even less so for it to occur as radically as it recently did. To name a particular case, before the health crisis, in higher education, only 19% of programs were aimed at distance learning, and 16% implemented blended learning at universities with a virtual approach (OCDE, 2015).

It is impossible not to recognize online education's advantages: instant communication, access to unlimited content, more effective data processing, among others. However, conditions, resources, and tools are not available to everyone, so the experience cannot be effective enough, as was originally suggested.

During the last two decades, Mexico has invested an important quantity of resources (financial, human, and institutional) to insert the technological component into teaching and learning processes. Starting with programs such as Enciclomedia, Habilidades Digitales para Todos, and finally Aprende 2.0, Mexican authorities have attempted to make information and communication technologies available to teachers and students in a relevant and pertinent manner to develop digital competencies.

Despite the undeniable progress regarding access and investment in education and digital infrastructure in Mexican schools, gaps, unfortunately, prevail, especially among areas of a lower socioeconomic status. As it is stated in the following table, the data provided by the Programme for International Student Assessment (PISA) assessment show us that there is a significant gap between schools: 5 out of every 10 students in Mexico have access to a computer for schoolwork, while the OECD's average is greater (89%). Concerning Mexican schools, those in a disadvantage condition only allow 2 out of every 10 students to use a computer. Regarding internet access, while the OECD's average determines that 9 out of every 10 students have a computer with internet access, in Mexico, only 7 out 10 have it. It is important to comparatively observe that between schools at an advantage and those at a disadvantage, the gaps grow alarmingly wider.

Currently, the pandemic has highlighted the Mexican education system's frailty, demonstrating an undeniable reality. Inequalities dependent on the area, locality and socioeconomic conditions prevail across the country despite the expansion and coverage of internet services undergone during the last few years. According to the 2018 statistical yearbook published by the Instituto Federal de Telecomunicaciones (Federal Telecommunication

Institute, IFT), Mexico City, along with Sonora, shares the highest number of citizens with a mobile broadband connection having 91 per every 100 citizens with access to it. They are followed by Baja California Sur (86), Quintana Roo (82), Baja California (82), and Yucatan (82). Last in the ranking are Chiapas (33), Oaxaca (42), and Guerrero (46). Regarding fixed-line internet connection, the national average shows that 51 out of every 100 households have internet access. In the country's capital, internet access is 96 for every 100 citizens, with the highest rank in the country. It is followed by Nuevo León (76), Querétaro (72), Baja California (70), and Jalisco; Chiapas (17), Oaxaca (22), and Tabasco (23) rank the lowest.

Table 1. *Percentage of Students with Access to Technology Resources at Their Schools*

<table>
<tr><td colspan="6">Students with a computer for schoolwork</td></tr>
<tr><td>OECD average</td><td>Average in Mexico</td><td colspan="2">Average in schools at an advantage</td><td colspan="2">Average in schools at a disadvantage</td></tr>
<tr><td rowspan="2">89%</td><td rowspan="2">56%</td><td>Mexico</td><td>24%</td><td>Mexico</td><td>88%</td></tr>
<tr><td>OECD</td><td>81%</td><td>OECD</td><td>95%</td></tr>
<tr><td colspan="6">Students with a computer with internet access</td></tr>
<tr><td>OECD average</td><td>Average in Mexico</td><td colspan="2">Average schools at an advantage</td><td colspan="2">Average schools at a disadvantage</td></tr>
<tr><td rowspan="2">95%</td><td rowspan="2">68%</td><td>Mexico</td><td>30%</td><td>Mexico</td><td>94%</td></tr>
<tr><td>OECD</td><td>90%</td><td>OECD</td><td>100%</td></tr>
</table>

Note: A school at a socioeconomic disadvantage is one with a socioeconomic background (that is, the average socioeconomic status of all students in the school) that score in the lowest quartile of PISA's economic, social, and cultural index for all schools in the country. Meanwhile, an advantaged school is one with a high socioeconomic background that can be found in the higher rankings of the economic, social, and cultural index.

Source: OECD, 2020.

Nevertheless, in order to take advantage of the online education brought about by the context of the pandemic, having a computer and internet access is not enough; good internet speed, a resource that is not available to all people and in all homes, is also relevant. As already emphasized in Reimers and Schleicher's (2020) report, "A framework to guide an education response to the COVID-19 pandemic of 2020," evidence provided by OECD PISA, shows that the majority of education systems were not prepared to offer online learning opportunities to the majority of students. This does not only highlight the differences between countries, but the growing gaps within each's socioeconomic groups as well. In Mexico, 94% of 15-year-old students with privileged backgrounds have internet connections in their homes, but only 29% of those from underprivileged backgrounds had access to it. In addition to this, some factors that may condition access to a high-quality online education are social context, race, ethnicity, area, type of institution or learning modality, and the parents' education, among others.

The current scenario implies even bigger challenges in comparison to the previous complex and adverse scenario, but it also brings opportunities. Having this in mind, we raise the following question: Will educational technologies aid in the democratization of access to education and reduction of social gaps, or will they have the opposite effect?

Just as Mancera, Serna, and Barrios (2020) argued, the pandemic has had an adverse effect on equal opportunity. An immediate effect is the cancellation of school. On the medium and long term, effects will be observable through the measure at which technological resources and support become equitably available to teachers.

As Lloyd (2020) highlighted, in normal times, these differences would be another piece in Mexico's mosaic of disparities, but during the COVID-19 pandemic the digital gap has been particularly harmful and generated far-reaching consequences, especially, in the education system. Limited access to ICTs affects students from preschool to university, by determining who has access to online education. In the higher levels of education, 55% of the students within the first income decile do not have a computer or internet access at home. Conversely, for the richest decile the number is only 2% according to National Income and Expenditure Survey or Encuesta Nacional de Ingresos y Gastos del Hogar (INEGI, 2018). On average, 18% of university students do not have access to the previously mentioned services, which means that one in five cannot attend online classes. In high school education, the gap is even wider: 81% of the people or students living in poverty do not have internet or a computer at home, compared to 3% of the student population that comes from more privileged households. Finally, on average 40% do not have access to ICT in their homes (INEGI, 2018).

It is impossible to say that the pandemic created a gap in the education system or that it generated the current educational disparities. The pandemic was the detonator of a problem rooted in the education system and in our society. ICT can be useful for the effective design and development of education policies that combat disparities, but they will not be the end-all of this phenomenon.

The Mexican education system has struggled to overcome the current challenges posed by public health issues. The analysis performed by Fernández, Herrera, Hernández, Nolasco, and de la Rosa (2020) states the following:

- The lack of adequate teacher training on the use of ICT for the every-day pedagogical experience.
- The "acquisition" of computers, laptops, tablets, and other kinds of technologies which were supposed to be distributed among teachers and a significant number of students, but instead represented an inadequate expense and represented several millions worth of fraud due to total absence, mismanagement, and lax control during the distribution of these resources, only a handful of students had access to them and to online education.
- A lackluster adaptation of the materials used during in-person classes to teach the subjects of different educational levels into a digital format suitable for online teaching.
- The lack of policies to address disparities in the access to internet for educational purposes faced by a very significant number of students in the country (only 39.1% of the population in rural areas has internet access according to the INEGI's 2018 National Survey on Availability and Use of Information Technologies in the Home).

This is why, facing this unprecedented situation requires the implementation of flexible and creative strategies that allow for a pedagogical and administrative adaptation of great scope. This represents a challenge but also an opportunity to move forward, though in a forceful and fast-tracked manner, with strategies that enable the teaching/learning process' response to current trends without neglecting the goal of achieving inclusive and quality education. Without a doubt, this scenario can be a starting point for the introduction of a new education system in Mexico.

The "Aprende en Casa" Program

The "Aprende en casa" (Learn at Home) program was the digital platform with learning resources designed and implemented by the Ministry of Education (SEP) with objective of helping students finish the 2019-2020 school cycle after schools closed due to the COVID-19 pandemic. This education program consists of recreating the textbooks' curricular content through public television broadcasts of pedagogical and recreational shows.

For the 2020-2021 cycle, SEP reinforced the program resulting in the creation of "Aprende en Casa II," which covered a larger number of contents and had wider national coverage as it was broadcast on new channels 24 hours a day, seven days a week. The program has been useful and helpful for students and parents to mitigate the learning deficits generated by confinement. One of the most innovative aspects of the program is the access to a platform that is available on any device and covers a wide range of the day's subjects according to the level of education. In order to encourage the students to stay in the program and increase their interest, SEP has had several character and celebrity appearances with the aim of creating content that is more recreational, attractive and interesting.

However, there are still areas of opportunity to explore in order to limit the gaps of disparity that prevail in our system and the access to ICT is widening. One of the most relevant issues is the lack of training teachers received to adapt the contents and class dynamic to the other modalities. Ensuring that teachers have the necessary digital skills is still a pending task for the authorities. There is no way to guarantee equal access to the acquisition of digital skills if the resources and training are only available for a few number of teachers.

In the same way, another current issue that has been identified by international organizations and academic institutions through the use of surveys and opinion-polls is the lack of motivation of students for online learning. The emotional state of students is an aspect of the confinement that grants consideration and will become a phenomenon with serious short, medium, and long-term effects. According to diverse qualitative studies (UNICEF, Tec de Monterrey, UIA, 2020), a significant number of students have expressed feeling sad, frustrated, angry, anxious, stressed, and weary, among other things. The COVID-19 pandemic is challenging the resilience of thousands of students and teachers in Mexico, the Mexican government will require a timely intervention in this area if they wish to prevent school desertion in the future.

As we have previously mentioned, our country does not have equal access to ICTs in both schools and homes. The "Aprende en Casa"[1] program only serves as a substitute for the lack of in-person classes. To achieve better results and close the gaps, schools need to invest on resources such as computer equipment, connectivity, and software, as well as training and planning to ease the transition of teachers and students into the new modality, and a way to monitor the results. Additionally, to reach the objective of reducing disparities, it is necessary to strengthen the relationships with private stakeholders, civil society organizations, foundations and international agencies under a collaborative model through which, the State allows contributions to the established milestones and reinforce the implementation of programs in an independent and objective manner using evidence.

In order to achieve an effective and appropriate digital education program it is necessary for the national educational system's stakeholders to have a certain degree of digitization and for classrooms to have the minimum resources necessary to implement the model equitably. Furthermore, in the future, the model should rely on an instructional design approach that allows teachers to generate more interaction, enabling communication between students and teachers and improving the teaching/learning process and the design of an appropriate evaluation model.

Recommendations

As a result of the current situation, the State's responsibility lies on the mitigation of social disparities and educational gaps derived from the effects of the pandemic, focusing on the most vulnerable sectors or populations. Disparities will increase as a result of the pandemic, generating effects that will greatly affect millions of girls, boys, and young people without the implementation of appropriate measures and programs. The response to this unprecedented crisis requires leadership, long-term vision, and coordination, as well as the political will to adopt public policy alternatives that mitigate the high economic and social costs coming from the pandemic. Therefore, we recommend the following:

- Develop educational policies that benefit girls, boys, and young people in vulnerable situations. The many faces of educational disparity negatively affect human development when it comes to access to opportunities, income, and improved work prospects. The Mexican education system shows an alarming tendency to perpetuate educational disparity as a result of the school setting students find themselves in, meaning that there is a dynamic concerning access to education that depends on socioeconomic status yielding predetermined consequences for the future. Low-income households and population sectors that are usually sidelined, must be assisted through compensatory programs meant to reduce the disparity gaps and guarantee quality education.

- Focus on the students' health and well-being promptly addressing the socio-emotional effects of this crisis on students constitutes a priority, as students from different levels of education are at risk of developing disorders. The shift in the dynamics and environments surrounding girls, boys, and young people have created disturbances and tension in the family, social, and school settings. As a result, it is essential for governments to develop workshops and spaces designed to help students cope and channel emotions commonly associated with crises through the appropriate techniques such as active listening, receptive attitudes, and sympathy. Special care must be taken regarding young people and adolescents, as they are particularly vulnerable to behavioral and emotional imbalances that may result in school desertion, domestic violence, drug use, or suicide.

- Devise a comprehensive strategy to reopen schools. Before this, it is important to mention that it will be difficult to plan for reopening without safety measures and the consent of teachers. If this is achieved, the government should consider the well-being of students and teachers as well as, infrastructure and necessary resources to ensure the safety of school in terms of compliance with sanitary and hygiene measures. For example, following social distancing guidelines would require having classes with only 10 to 12 students, which is impossible for many schools in the country.

- Eventually, close the digital gap. It is fundamental to double-down on the efforts to guarantee access to technology and reduce the digital gap, especially in marginalized and vulnerable homes. Additionally, the digital gap will have a negative effect on gender disparity, as women have more limited access to ICT than men. The several effects of this health and economic crisis will exacerbate the reality faced by girls and women of all ages in Mexico: A clear gender gap regarding the access to ICTs which represents a barrier that inhibits their full development and future inclusion in work spheres. As such, guaranteeing access to educational platforms containing large collections of educational resources is fundamental.

- Secure the levels of public expenditure for education. It is customary to perform budget cuts to public expenditure during crises in order to divert funds towards economic recovery. Education represents an investment for governments, not an expenditure. Therefore, it is vital to maintain the levels of public expenditure to reinforce educational progress and mitigate the effects of the health crisis.

Final Thoughts

According to Fernando Reimers y Andreas Schleicher (2020), the effects of the COVID-19 pandemic will seriously hinder the learning of students and will affect at least one entire generation. Easing their impact will greatly depend on the actions taken by educational administrative authorities of all levels and the support of private social and academic stakeholders.

Now more than ever, the relevant education system stakeholders including students, teachers, supervisors, school principals, authorities, and parents must be ready to face the changes to the teaching process in the next few years.

This challenge will not be easy, as Mexico deals with economic, social, and educational gaps that have been very difficult to close in the past. The current context is filled with uncertainty and challenges us to reflect on the education we want and will have to define, design, and implement so that it serves the purpose of helping students competently deal with current challenges. On top of this, the role stakeholders have in education must be reconsidered to enable equitable education on a short, medium and long term basis.

Everything must be done to prevent a generational educational catastrophe as a result of this public health phenomenon that has negatively impacted our social habits, economic conditions, as well as personal and professional activities. The decisions made by authorities, particularly educational authorities, will have implications for the childhood and youth in Mexico. Now more than ever, we have to invest in the future of the new generations that will become the driving force of growth and progress in our country in the medium and long term.

The current health crisis has shed light on the core issues of education and has shown us that the inclusion of ICTs may be one of the necessary conditions to achieve equity. If the country suffers a setback, it will be very difficult to close the prevailing gaps of disparity through a gradual embrace of the distance learning modality in the medium and long term.

It is fundamental that the guideline of the Mexican government in the coming years must focus on strengthening equity to achieve educational quality as the pillars of education policy. Any programs, policies or interventions will be more effective if we prioritize educational and technical criteria during the improvement of the education model. Without this, improving the quality and closing the gaps of disparity will remain a wish but not a reality for millions of Mexican students.

Only time, and its unavoidable effects and consequences will tell us if Mexico had the vision, flexibility, ability, and resources to face the current situation as both a challenge and an unprecedented opportunity for education. Therefore, NEM is being challenged with the objective of achieving educational equity and the fundamental improvement of the education system which is more urgent than ever before. In an international and national context of never-ending crises and high uncertainty, where paradigms are constantly shifting, mainly due to the accelerated technological advancements, education must transform and adapt strategically, appropriately, and promptly.

Bibliography

Blanco, E. (2011). Los límites de la escuela. Educación, desigualdad y aprendizaje en México. México: El Colegio de México, Centro de Estudios Sociológicos. Retrieved from: https://www.ses.unam.mx/curso2013/pdf/BlancoEmilio.pdf

Bracho, T. (1995). Distribución y desigualdad educativa en México. *Revista Estudios Sociológicos,* 8 (37), 25-37.

El Colegio de México. (2018). *Desigualdades en México.* México: El Colegio de México—Red de Estudios sobre Desigualdades.

Esquivel, G. (2015). *Desigualdad extrema en México.* México: Oxfam.

Evans, David. (2020). How Will COVID-19 Affect Women and Girls in Low- and Middle-Income Countries? Retrieved from: www.cgdev.org/blog/how-will-covid-19-affect-women-and-girls-low-and-middle-income-countries

Giorguli, S., Vargas, E., Salinas, V., Hubert, C., and Potter, J. (2010). La dinámica demográfica y la desigualdad educativa en México. *Estudios Demográficos y Urbanos,* 25 (1), 7-44.

Fernández, M., Herrera, L. Hernández, D., Nolasco, R. and De la Rosa, R. (2020). Lecciones del COVID para el sistema educativo mexicano. *Nexos. Distancia por tiempos.* Blog de educación.

Hutchinson, P., Mirzoyants, A., and Leyton, A. (2019). Empowering youth for social change through the Shujaaz multimedia platform in Kenya. Retrieved from: www.shujaazinc.com/wp-content/uploads/2020/01/Empowering-youth-for-social-change-through-the-Shujaaz-multimedia-platform-in-Kenya.pdf

Instituto Federal de Telecomunicaciones. (2018). Anuario Estadístico 2018. Retrieved from: http://www.ift.org.mx/sites/default/files/contenidogeneral/estadisticas/anuarioestadistico2018-111018.pdf

Instituto Nacional de Estadística y Geografía. (2018). Encuesta Nacional de Ingresos y Gastos de los Hogares 2018. Retrieved from: https://www.inegi.org.mx/programas/enigh/nc/2018/

Lustig, N., Martinez, V., Sanz, F. and Younger, S. D. (2020). The impact of

COVID-19 lockdowns and expanded social assistance on inequality, poverty and mobility in Argentina, Brazil, Colombia and Mexico. Retrieved from: http://repec.tulane.edu/RePEc/ceq/ceq92.pdf

Mancera, C., Serna, L. y Barrios, M. (2020). Pandemia: Maestros, tecnología y desigualdad. Available at: https://educacion.nexos.com.m/?p=2286

Martínez, F. (1992). La desigualdad educativa en México. *Revista Latinoamericana de Estudios Educativos*, 22 (2), 59-120.

Muñoz-Izquierdo, C. (1996). *Origen y consecuencias de las desigualdades educativas*. Investigaciones realizadas en América Latina sobre el problema. México: Fondo de Cultura Económica.

Organización para la Cooperación y el Desarrollo Económicos. (2015). E-Learning in Higher Education in Latin America. Retrieved from: https://www.oecd.org/publications/e-learning-in-higher-education-in-latin-america-9789264209992-en.htm

Programa de Naciones Unidad para el Desarrollo. (2020). Desarrollo humano y Covid-19 en México: desafíos para una recuperación sostenible. Retrieved from: www.mx.undp.org/content/mexico/es/home/library/poverty/desarrollo-humano-y-covid-19-en-mexico-.html

Schmelkes, S. (1997). *La calidad en la educación primaria: un estudio de caso.* Ciudad de México: Fondo de Cultura Económica.

Schmelkes, S. (2010). Indígenas rurales, migrantes, urbanos: una educación equivocada, otra educación posible, en Marchesi, Álvaro y Margarita Poggi (eds.), *Presente y futuro de la educación iberoamericana*, Madrid: AECID.

Solís, P. (2012). Social mobility in Mexico. Trends, recent findings and research challenges. TRACE, 62, 7-20.

Székely, M. (1995). Aspectos de la desigualdad en México. *El trimestre económico*, 62 (246), 201-243.

Rothe, D., Lagaay, M., Gallinetti, J. and Campbell, L. (2014). Young lives on lockdown: The impact of Ebola on children and communities in Liberia. Retrieved from: https://resourcecentre.savethechildren.net/node/8708/pdf/ih-liberia_ebola_interim_report-final-io-eng-dec14_1.pdf

COVID-19 and Mexico's Economic Outlook

Juan Carlos Baker and Rosángel Hernández

Introduction: How the Pandemic Found Mexico

At the time of writing this piece, the world has coexisted with the COVID-19 for more than 13 months. However, there is still few certainties about it, and with a few notable exceptions (such as New Zealand, Taiwan, South Korea, Vietnam), most governments haven't had success in controlling its spread. As never before in the history of mankind, human, technological, and economic resources are being poured to find a vaccine against this disease.

In the midst of all the uncertainty surrounding COVID-19 there is one thing clear: closing the economy and imposing strict mobility restrictions on the population, as mechanisms to prevent its spread—despite the results it may offer in the immediate term—is unsustainable in the long term and could even be counterproductive. In the case of Mexico, this reality is even more striking.

Mexico began 2020 with a very complex economic outlook. In 2019, the economy fell by -0.3%, and several important indicators on the overall performance of economic activity, such as construction, gross fixed investment, and manufacturing production showed also significant setbacks in that year (See Table 1).

Table 1. *Mexico 2019: Selected Economic Indicators*
(Real percentage change compared to previous year)

Indicator	2019
GDP	**-0.3**
Secondary activities	**-1.7**
– Mining	-5.1
– Construction	-4.9
– Manufacturing industries	0.4
Gross Fixed Investment	**-4.9**

Source: INEGI, 2020a, 2020b.

In line with 2019 results, at the beginning of 2020, international organizations and rating agencies estimated that the Mexican economy could grow between 0.7% and 1.3% in 2020. Naturally, the COVID-19 pandemic worsened those forecasts. It took Mexico from a difficult economic context to an even more complex scenario. Thus, the country suffered a double blow: on the one hand, the shutdown of the Mexican economy itself, and on the other, with the shutdown of the rest of the world, Mexico's main sources of income were cut off: international trade (equivalent to 70% of Gross Domestic Product, GDP) and tourism (8.7% of GDP). In addition, although not directly related to COVID-19, the fall in oil prices severely affected Mexican finances.

Understandably, the fragile situation of the Mexican economy didn't go unnoticed by international organizations. At the beginning of March 2020, the United Nations Conference on Trade and Development (UNCTAD) estimated that, due to its high interdependence with international markets, Mexico was among the fifteen economies that would be most affected by the commercial impact of COVID-19. UNCTAD estimated that the disruptions caused in supply chains that depended on China would affect around $1.3 billion USD of Mexico's exports (2020).

During the following months, it was common to see increasingly pessimistic forecasts for the Mexican economy. For example, the World Bank (2020) predicted a -7.5% drop and the International Monetary Fund (IMF, 2020) a -10.5% fall for Mexico's GDP in 2020. Even the reports of the Mexican Ministry of Finance and Public Credit (2020) acknowledged the difficult economic context for the country.

Considering this outlook, this text analyzes the impact caused by COVID-19 in Mexico during the first half of 2020. The objective is to try to foresee some of the areas in which the pandemic will have long-term effects in the country. To this end, we divide this text into two main sections according to the two major moments we identified in the development of the COVID-19 pandemic in Mexico: the first moment, when the magnitude and economic impact that COVID-19 was causing in the world and especially in Mexico began to be understood; and the second moment in which the public debate on how to move forward intensified. Finally, the conclusions point out some aspects that should be considered going forward to support the country's recovery.

The First Moment: Understanding the Cost of the Pandemic

As the pandemic progressed, it became evident that a vaccine would be needed to control it. Also, it became clear that keeping the economy closed for a long period of time and imposing mobility restrictions on the population were unsustainable and could be counterproductive.

Then, an article published by *The Economist* (2020) showed how keeping the economy closed, together with restrictions on people's mobility, could affect considerably more lives than it saves in three main ways:

i. Increasing extreme poverty. Closing the economy or partially reducing economic activity eliminates sources of employment for thousands of people who would suddenly be left with no opportunity to generate income. This could have serious consequences on the economy of lower-income families who typically live on day-to-day with little or no savings. Considering this situation, ideally, governments should supplement, through social policy, the income of the most vulnerable population. However, it is clear that governments could not help them all. For example, in sub-Saharan Africa, the poorest people have only a 4% chance of receiving government assistance in normal times. Thus, in times of COVID-19, 420 million people could fall into extreme poverty.

ii. Opening the door for outbreaks of diseases other than COVID-19. Quarantines have prevented the regular deployment of World Health Organization (WHO) vaccination programs, which could lead to the emergence of new outbreaks of other diseases with high mortality rates, such as malaria, AIDS, or measles. According to estimates by *The Economist*, in Africa, 140 children are at risk of dying for every death prevented from COVID-19.

iii. Increasing mortality from other diseases, due to the lack of attention by health systems absorbed by COVID-19. For instance, delaying cancer consultations in England for six months would imply the loss of 40% of the life years gained by treating an equivalent number of COVID-19 patients.

Two valuable lessons can be drawn from this information. First, considering that it is difficult for government programs to reach all those in need during "normal times," during the COVID-19 pandemic it is critical that those people in economic vulnerability count with the alternatives to continue their economic activity. Second, the health, economic and social security systems must be prepared to face new outbreaks of COVID-19 or other epidemics, in order to prevent that more people are at risk of falling into extreme poverty.

In Mexico's case, the COVID-19 pandemic has deepened the economic recession, especially since the second quarter of 2019. As Table 2 shows, the impact of COVID-19, which is reflected especially in 2020's second quarter (II), has been more critical in secondary activities, which comprise manufacturing and construction industries, as well as in tertiary activities, where service and trade activities are concentrated, both key sectors for the Mexican economy.

A recent article published by Gerardo Esquivel (2020) addresses that the most critical effects of COVID-19's economic impact can be comprised in two interrelated concepts: employment and poverty. In his analysis, he establishes three aspects of the country's current scenario that reflects this situation:

Table 2. *GDP 2019-2020, by Quarter*
(Real % change compared to the same period of the previous year)

Concept	**2019**					**2020**[P]		
	I	**II**	**III**	**IV**	**Annual**	**I**	**II**	**6 months**
GDP	**1.1**	**-1.1**	**-0.4**	**-0.7**	**-0.3**	**-1.3**	**-18.7**	**-10.1**
Primary activities	1.6	-1.2	1.9	-0.3	0.4	0.9	-0.5	0.2
Secondary activities	-0.2	-3.0	-1.4	-2.0	-1.7	-2.6	-25.7	-14.1
Tertiary activities	1.6	-0.3	-0.1	-0.2	0.2	-0.7	-16.2	-8.5

Source: INEGI, 2020a.

- From March to June 2020, 1.1 million formal jobs were lost, which represented a 5.4% reduction in the total number of jobs registered in the Mexican Social Security Institute (IMSS). The bulk of the loss occurred in the months of April and May, in which 900,000 jobs were lost.
- The loss of jobs has been concentrated among workers at the lowest income levels: 83.7% of all job losses correspond to workers earning between 1 and 2 minimum wages.

- The most affected sectors have been agriculture (-11.5%), construction (-10.1%), and the service industry (-8.6%). These three sectors account for 60% of all job losses during the pandemic.

The concentration of job losses among the lowest wage levels leads to the next distressing element of the pandemic in Mexico: the increase in poverty. The National Council for the Evaluation of Social Development Policy (2020) projects that with only a 5.3% decrease in GDP, between 6.1 and 10.7 million people could fall into extreme poverty in 2020. Even more worrying, it is important to consider that the reality is likely to exceed these estimates since, as we know now, the decrease in GDP will most likely be well above the 5.3% estimated by CONEVAL.

After the deep economic crisis of 1994 and 2009, eight years needed to elapse before pre-crisis levels of food and material poverty recovered (Villanueva, 2020). This points at vulnerability economic and sanitary crises provoked by the COVID-19 may generate, including erasing the social progress achieved in the last decade, compromising the capacity of the business sector and households to recover and even to reduce the potential of the Mexican economy as a whole.

However, the worst mistake that we could do is to think that, without the pandemic, Mexico would not face economic hardship. COVID-19 has not created new problems, but rather it has brought visibility to the existing structural problems that have affected our society for a long time, and that unfortunately have not been addressed through several administrations: weak health systems, deepening income disparity, a growing informal economy, and work schemes that produce further precarity to workers' environment, just to name a few examples.

The Second Moment: How to Move Forward

According to the Harvard University method for crisis management, a basic principle is that, when facing a crisis, leaders have two main responsibilities: (1) address the immediate problem; and (2) diminish the effects. The former is the more urgent, but the latter is what minimize the long—term negative consequences.

This has become one of the key elements of Mexico's national discussion: What should we do to minimize the economic impact of the COVID-19?

Inevitably, the debate has polarized the public opinion among those who consider that health must be the driving priority over the economy, and those who think exactly the opposite. However, this is a false dilemma. In reality, one cannot exist without the other, e.g., saving lives is what will save the economy, and thus efforts must be implemented simultaneously in both fronts.

On the economic side, a large part of governments has decided to introduce countercyclical measures, injecting extraordinary amounts of cash into the economy through fiscal stimulus. In the United States, for example, Congress has voted stimulus for more than 3 trillion U.S. dollars, whereas the European Union approved a stimulus package worth 750 billion euros.

Mexico is among the very few countries that have not recurred to these measures, even for Latin American standards, as shown in Table 2. Fiscal stimulus and spending in Mexico are barely 1% of the GDP, while the average in Latin America equals to 3.9% of the GDP. However, some renowned economists such as J. Stiglitz y H. Rashid (2020) have argued that it is not clear that an aggressive fiscal strategy may be the most adequate response to the economic crisis caused by the COVID-19.

Table 3. *Spending, Fiscal, and Liquidity Measures Against COVID-19in Latin America* (% GDP)

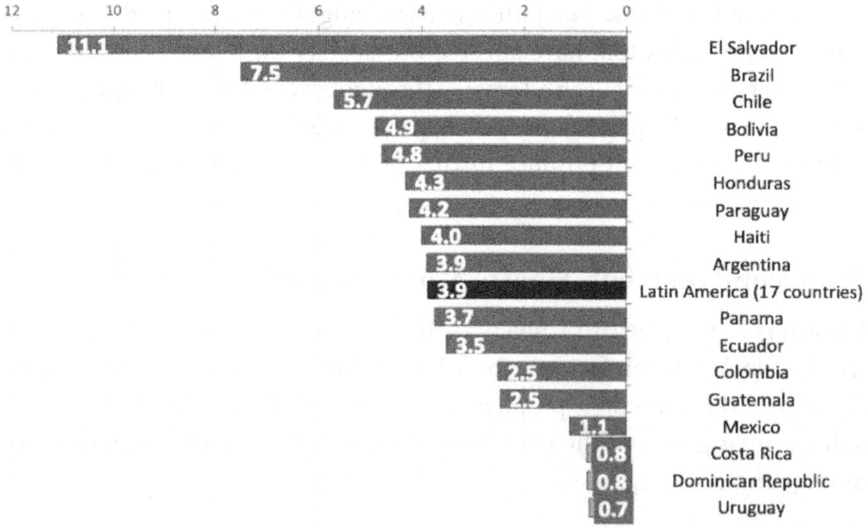

Source: ECLAC, 2020.

It is important to consider that there could be many ways to support the economy without undertaking more debt or further spending—for example, financing low interests rates for companies to maintain workers registered in the Mexican Institute of Social Security (IMSS); establishing a tax deferral regime on manufacturing exporting companies, at which over 2.7 million Mexicans work; and creating fiscal and credit schemes that assist small and medium companies to better absorb the consumption fall without laying off workers, among others.

Moreover, it is fundamental to design focalized strategies for those sectors more exposed and at risk. Many of them are found in the services sector, especially tourism (which employs over 4.4 million workers in Mexico) and recreational services, including movie theaters, sports and concerts, and others. Finally, in order to increase the resilience of this sector in the case of future contingencies, a strategy aimed at recovering consumers' confidence and consumers' safety is urgent.

It is necessary for Mexico to guarantee that it will continue to be a reliable and trustable host for investments and international trade. The entry into force of the United States-Mexico-Canada Agreement (USMCA) on July 2020 is a major contributing factor for economy stability in Mexico, and its context becomes even more relevant in the light of two aspects: because, on the one hand, the USMCA fits nicely in the current context where regional value chains are preferred, particularly when other economic activities in Mexico do not have an optimist perspective; and second, because the USMCA will promote more economic integration in North America against a complex international environment.

However, this will only happen if Mexico generates an environment of legal certainty to do business in the country, coupled with the promotion of public policies that favor the companies' productivity and their technological sophistication. The cancellation of foreign investments (such as a brewery in Mexicali[1]), together with other signals of potential changes to the legal framework (as it was the case with recent decisions regarding renewable energies[2]), will continue to erode investors' confidence in the country, which

1 In March 2020, after a public consultation, Mexico's government cancelled the construction of a *Constellation Brands* brewery in Mexicali. The decision to cancel a project which had a 70% progress was widely criticized by the business community in the country.

2 On April 29th, 2020, the National Center for Energy Control (CENACE) published

will in turn augment the vulnerability of the country towards future sanitary and economic contingencies.

If an environment that promotes investors' confidence is created, the negative economic consequences of the COVID-19 can indeed be limited. Families would be able to spend more and apply for credit to acquire properties and more durable goods if the perceived risk of losing their jobs and companies is not high; furthermore, companies would invest in new businesses or reinforce existing ones if there are adequate incentives from the government to reactivate the economy.

Conclusions

After the COVID-19, the world and Mexico will be different in several dimensions. Globally, we will see the acceleration of discussion and adoption of new public policies, especially in the social realm. For example, there will be a growing debate regarding the adoption of a universal basic income and fully paid mandatory sickness leave, especially in middle-income countries.

Similarly, it is important to consider that the research, development and manufacturing of medicines and drugs would be subject to pressures from governments, not only to incentivize the establishment of domestic industries, but also to demand a larger participation in the definition of research objectives and priorities. This last point could be viable considering that governments will want to strengthen the sanitary structure and safety of their systems, in order to demonstrate to their societies that said governments have the knowledge and capacity to address any future contingencies. It is also likely that some governments seek to regulate pharmaceutical companies with stricter protocols, which would inevitably have implications on the structure of the industry and its organization.

Mexico must conduct a profound assessment of its health system. COVID-19 has made painfully clear how insufficient the current infrastructure is, but it also demonstrated how vulnerable the average Mexican citizen is: it has

---

a decree, whose objective allegedly was to guarantee the efficiency, quality, reliability and continuity of the national electric system. In essence, this decree suspended the operational tests of 17 solar and wind electrical centrals. Following such decree, on May 15th, an additional decree was published by the Ministry of Energy where a more prominent role was given to the Federal Electricity Commission (CFE) to supply the Mexican electricity market, affecting current investments in the sector and discouraging future investment opportunities.

been demonstrated that the high rate of diseases such as diabetes (10% of the population), obesity (highest world rate after the U.S.) and high-blood pressure (18% of the population) have increased the exposure of Mexico's population to the COVID-19 (Eschenbacher and Barrera, 2020).

Economically, Mexico must prepare itself to coexist with the pandemic. There are already several companies operating under the strictest sanitary regulations. Communication and sharing of best practices among the business community in the country will be key in the next few months. Moreover, as long as we do not have a COVID-19 vaccine, there will be incentives to impede the possible physical interactions, digitalizing as many activities as possible, not only in the economic realm, but practically in every activity that we could possibly think of, from medical consultation to legal and government permits.

Facing the several deep transformation processes already on their way, and the many others that we can anticipate in the short term, it is fundamental that government, private industry, and all society stakeholders join efforts to generate strategies that multiply the positive effects in health and economics. Finally, Mexico should also work towards harmonize and align its responses with those of its USMCA partners in addressing the most urgent questions of the pandemic, thus it will be able to detonate further economic activity that would facilitate the recovery of the country.

Bibliography

CONEVAL. (2020). La crisis sanitaria generada por la COVID-19 y sus consecuencias económicas ponen en riesgo avances en desarrollo social. Retrieved from: https://www.coneval.org.mx/Evaluacion/IEPSM/Paginas/Politica_Social_COVID-19.aspx

ECLAC. (2020). Enfrentar los efectos cada vez mayores del COVID-19 para una reactivación con igualdad: nuevas proyecciones. Retrieved from: https://www.cepal.org/sites/default/files/presentation/files/final_200714_version_revisada_ab-ppt_informe_covid_5_15_julio.pdf

Esquivel, G. (2020). Los impactos económicos de la pandemia en México. México: Banxico. Retrieved from: https://www.banxico.org.mx/

publicaciones-y-prensa/articulos-y-otras-publicaciones/%7BD442A596-6F43-D1B5-6686-64A2CF2F371B%7D.pdf

S. Eschenbacher and A. Barrera. (2020). With obesity and diabetes epidemic, Mexico braces for coronavirus. Reuters. Retrieved from: https://news.trust.org/item/20200326195209-a8sl7

IMF. (2020). Actualización de las perspectivas de la economía mundial. Retrieved from: https://www.imf.org/es/Publications/WEO/Issues/2020/06/24/WEOUpdateJune2020

INEGI. (2020a). Producto Interno Bruto de México durante el segundo trimestre de 2020. Retrieved from: https://www.inegi.org.mx/contenidos/saladeprensa/boletines/2020/pib_pconst/pib_pconst2020_08.pdf

INEGI. (2020b). Indicador Mensual de la Inversión Fija Bruta en México durante diciembre de 2019. Retrieved from: https://www.inegi.org.mx/contenidos/saladeprensa/boletines/2020/imfbcf/imfbcf2020_03.pdf

SHCP. (2020). Informes sobre la Situación Económica, las Finanzas Públicas y la Deuda Pública al segundo trimestre de 2020. Retrieved from: https://www.gob.mx/cms/uploads/attachment/file/566777/Comunicado_No._062.pdf

Stiglitz, J. and Rashid, H. (2020). Which economic stimulus work? Project Syndicate. Retrieved from: https://www.project-syndicate.org/commentary/stimulus-policies-must-benefit-real-economy-not-financial-speculation-by-joseph-e-stiglitz-and-hamid-rashid-2020-06

The Economist. (2020). Lifting lockdowns: the when, why and how. Retrieved from: https://www.economist.com/leaders/2020/05/23/lifting-lockdowns-the-when-why-and-how

UNCTAD. (2020). Coronavirus outbreak has cost global value chains $50 billion in exports. Retrieved from https://unctad.org/en/pages/newsdetails.aspx?OriginalVersionID=2297

Villanueva, D. (31 May 2020). Con ingresos bajos, 38 millones en el país antes del Covid: Inegi. La Jornada. Retrieved from: https://www.jor

nada.com.mx/ultimas/economia/2020/05/31/con-ingresos-bajos-38-millones-en-el-pais-antes-del-covid-inegi-9919.html

World Bank. (2020). Perspectivas económicas mundiales: América Latina y el Caribe. Retrieved from: http://pubdocs.worldbank.org/en/657071588788309322/Global-Economic-Prospects-June-2020-Regional-Overview-LAC-SP.pdf

What Happens in Mexican Prisons? A Review of the COVID-19 Pandemic Effects

Carol Aceval

The current world health crisis has increased the perception of the vulnerabilities that afflict Mexico. Just like a sick body, our country deeply resents its weakness and increasingly aches as a result of any stimulus. In areas such as security and justice, placing special emphasis on our penitentiary system, Mexico has responded towards COVID-19 with an excessive use of pre-trial detention throughout the years.

Throughout 2020, the COVID-19 pandemic has given us many lessons. One of them is that our penitentiary facilities cannot withstand the current health contingency, and without immediate change, will not withstand the future. The irrational use of prison, as a precautionary measure during trial or as a sanction after conviction, will continue to result in issues such as overpopulation, overcrowding and human rights violations for those facing the Mexican justice systems.

The world has over 11 million people in prison, and about 102 countries reported prison overcrowding levels over 110% (Penal Reform International, 2020). There were 210, +287 people under custody by June 2020; these people were held in 295 penitentiary facilities, and 118 of them were facing serious overcrowding issues. In addition to states such as New York and New Jersey in the U.S.A., countries like Finland (which has the lowest rates of incarceration in Europe) have become blueprints for decreasing prison population. Contrary to them, Mexico's numbers have not significantly decreased in the last years despite efforts (See Graph 1).

Given these population levels, the penitentiary system faces the COVID-19 pandemic while dealing with issues such as: space shortage, failed social reinsertion strategies, the so-called "revolving prison door," human rights violations, lack of financial resources, and manpower, among others. All this is in addition to the health crisis that mainly affects vulnerable groups, especially people under custody (Corte Interamericana de Derechos Humanos, 2020).

Graph 1. *Incarcerated Population Rate per Each 100,000 citizens in Mexico* 2000 – 2020

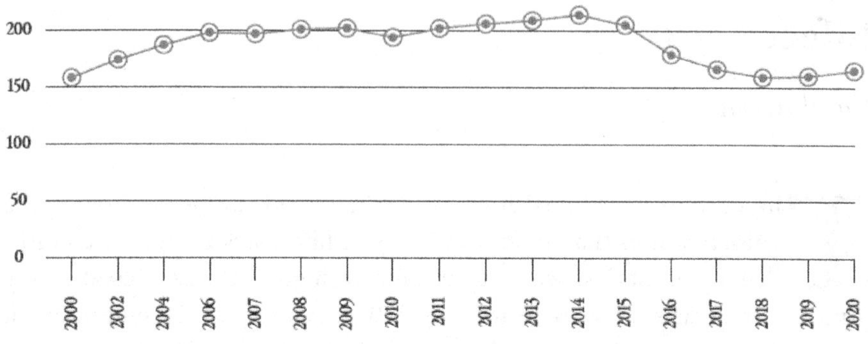

Source: OADPRS, 2020.

Excess and Generalization of Imprisonment: A Mexican Reality

According to the World Health Organization (WHO), imprisoned people are more vulnerable to the COVID-19 pandemic. This is due to the prolonged periods of confinement in which they live. Additionally, jails can become a source of infection, amplifying, and propagating contagious diseases beyond the facility. Due to this, health of people with justice system involvement in prison should be considered of paramount importance for public health (World Health Organization, 2020), considering that being in confinement increases the chances of higher case rates since people in prisons often come from places with higher poverty rates and marginalization where they could have been exposed to transmissible diseases, a lackluster diet, and limited access to quality healthcare (Penal Reform International, 2020).

What has led to this situation in the national penitentiary system? To answer this question, we must look back to the aspirations of the 2008 constitutional reform that came up due, then, to the foreseeable problems of excessive and generalized imprisonment. The Open Society Justice Initiative assessed Mexico's prisons as inadequate, exorbitant, unjust, and costly (Open Society Institute, 2004). As a response, Mexico implemented a new penal justice system and a new National System of Public Safety (Sistema Nacional de Seguridad Pública) that would meet the relevant international criteria. This new system favored the presumption of innocence and the application of specific measures to reduce pretrial detention.

In order to depressurize the prison system, these two measures needed to be implemented by June 2016, at the latest. Today, we can say that implementing and maintaining these changes have been a real challenge. Nowadays, we are still in the midst of a great conundrum when it comes to the excessive use of imprisonment. This has been magnified and further complicated due to the pandemic and its short, medium, and long-term effects.

The constitutional reform general provisions, previously mentioned, point out that this system would favor the presumption of innocence. This way, the accused would be recognized as a subject of rights and not the object of an investigation. Likewise, the transformation of the penitentiary system was planned in terms of social reinsertion axles: jobs, training, education, culture, and sports. On top of this, it is important to reflect upon the lesson and challenge posed by COVID-19 in a constitutional reform that is not yet effective for the purpose it was created. An example can be found in the 2020 Rule of Law Index (Estado de Derecho, 2020) where, in its penal justice system, Mexico holds 119th place out of 128 countries (The World Justice Project, 2020).

The Mexican model employed before the reform had a limited view of what could happen when someone face criminal proceedings. The classifications established in the penal procedural laws of federal and states would determine if a person could be submitted to pretrial detention or have the possibility of posting bail, thus facing the legal process in freedom before being sentenced. This caused an excessive use of prison, turning it into an early sentence. As this became the rule instead of the exception, it contradicted the criterion of the Inter-American Commission on Human Rights (2013), which had found it in "violation" to the pro-homine principle and in contradiction to Article 7.3 of the American Convention on Human Rights.

The 2011 Constitutional Reform regarding human rights, the issuing of the National Code of Penal Proceedings (Código Nacional de Procedimientos Penales) in 2014, and the 2016 National Penal Enforcement Law (Ley Nacional de Ejecución Penal) can be added to the list of legislative advances. They all facilitated one of the most sought-after changes of the penal justice system: imprisonment as the exception, the ultima ratio. This way, people could be treated as innocent until proven otherwise, avoiding the violation of human rights and seeking alternatives to deprivation of liberty that would aim to depressurize an overpopulated criminal system. Having this in mind, Sergio García Ramirez (2019) rightfully points out that pretrial detention constitutes a contradiction to the proclamation that oversees procedural law since the end of the eighteenth century, where a person is presumed innocent until they receive a guilty verdict.

Nonetheless, 2019 represented a noticeable setback: presumption of innocence and other attempts to solve the overcrowding issues in prisons were not enough to stop the "counter-reformation" of the 19th constitutional article. This widened the list of informal pretrial detention crimes. However, the Inter-American Court of Human Rights determined in the cases of Suárez Rosero Vs. Ecuador (1997) and López Álvarez Vs. Honduras (2006), that pretrial detention should not solely be based on the offence of which a person stands accused or the gravity of such, as they are not enough to justify imprisonment, and they could even be equated to an early sentence. Notwithstanding this, Mexico decided to bet in favor of pretrial detention even without evidence suggesting that criminal policy restricting personal liberty has any effect on reducing crime or violence or solving any public safety concerns (Comisión Interamericana de Derechos Humanos, 2013).

Said reform was based on argumentative fallacies, which claimed that doing this would increase safety and reduce the high rates of criminal activity in the country. Yet a year later, it has only yielded a higher number of imprisoned people who are awaiting trial. Even more worrying, there have been talks of a new wave of reforms, including some that contemplate pretrial detention for all crimes. As María Novoa (2020) accurately points out, Mexico is in a complex and dangerous situation that could even worsen safety within domestic territory.

Without doubt, such a limited precautionary model in the country has its drawbacks. In 2008, Mexico had a prison population of 219,574 people, while by June 2020, this number was around 210,000. This is proof of a consistent overpopulation and exploitation problem in an ineffective and expeditious system. Twelve years after Article 20, Section B, paragraph I, on the presumption of innocence principle was granted its constitutional status in Mexico, 85,265 individuals with justice system involvement are still in prison and waiting to be sentenced (OADPRS, 2020).

People In Custody: A Population at Risk

Now, it is essential for us to analyze the profile of people entering penitentiary facilities to understand the unrestrained use of prisons in Mexico. In 2018,

99,445 people were admitted into a state penitentiary facility, out of which 73.9% were admitted for the first time, meaning they were not repeat offenders. On top of this, 39.5% of the people were admitted due to alleged robbery charges and 14.4% due to alleged drug-dealing charges. Additionally, over 50% of people in prison were in for charges that could not be considered serious; moreover, 40.2% were between the ages of 18 and 29 and 38.2% only had secondary schooling. In this same year, 103,820 people were released from state penitentiary facilities; 5.6% of them were acquitted, and 1.8% had their sentence revoked (INEGI, 2019). It is worth asking ourselves if people being admitted into penitentiary facilities are, in fact, a big safety concern for our country, and whether they are really endangering our streets.

Furthermore, regarding the conditions of confinement in prisons, we may conclude that they are not the most favorable. The most recent national prison monitoring diagnostic of Comisión Nacional de los Derechos Humanos, or CNDH (2019), revealed that 183 or 33.3% of the facilities visited were overpopulated, and 32.24% showed signs of overcrowding (areas that were considerably past their capacity). To this day, in the midst of the pandemic, the State of Mexico stands out with a relative overpopulation of 117.88% (OADPRS, 2020).

It is worth pointing out that one of the most relevant findings of the 2019 National Diagnosis of Penitentiary Supervision (Diagnóstico Nacional de Supervisión Penitenciaria, 2019) highlighted the shortcomings of the health services inside these institutions. Out of 32.79% evaluated facilities that were under the charge of state authority, 26.78% were deficient when it came to practical conditions and the hygiene of medical facilities.

What is concerning in today's context is the evidence by the CNDH's Special Report, which shows the measures taken by penitentiary facilities to provide emergency healthcare for Sars-Cov2 (COVID-19). The report points out that "…the present contingency reached and surpassed the measures dictated by healthcare authorities for the prevention of the spread within penitentiary facilities in the country, transforming it into a scenario with the following shortcomings: materials, equipment, medicine, and infrastructure. All this is in addition to overcrowding, unfit living conditions due to deficiencies and lack of hygiene, as well as insufficient access to clean water and sanitation, and the invisible needs of vulnerable groups inside the prisons" (CNDH, 2020).

Graph 2. *Overpopulated Facilities in Mexico*

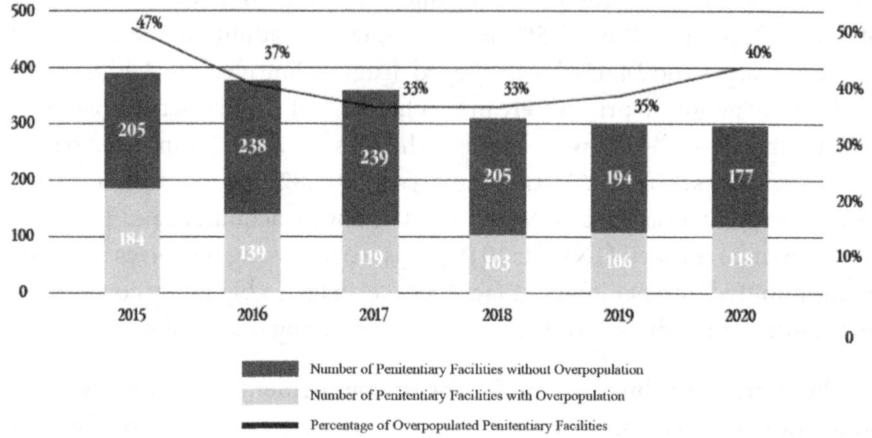

Source: Prepared by the author based on data from Cuaderno Mensual de Estadística Penitenciaria Nacional (National Monthly Penitentiary Statistic Notebook), June 2020.

It is obvious that the described scenario is a time bomb. A note published by the *New York Times* highlights that if spreading coronavirus were be deliberated, a typical Latin American or Caribbean jail would be the perfect space, due to their conditions. Consequently "reducing penitentiary population is crucial to avoid a general contagion inside the prison and the rest of society" (Acebes, 2020). This issue should have been contemplated and prevented many years ago and not when the effects of the pandemic are at their height. The invisibility of people under custody is taking its toll on the present, not just for the authorities in charge of custody but for the population as a whole.

It is interesting to see the monitoring that non-governmental organizations have done regarding the population under custody and the impacts of COVID-19. According to Así Legal (2020), a non-profit organization, 2,563 cases of COVID-19 had been reported within the Mexican penitentiary system by August 4th, 2020, of which 2,189 were people in custody, as well as 374 who were custodians or staff. Unfortunately, 193 people in custody and 49 custodians and staff have died as a result of COVID-19. Comparatively, the National Monitoring for COVID-19 in Penitentiary Facilities, performed by CNDH, showed that by July 14th there were 1,739 confirmed cases, 167 deaths, and 396 unconfirmed cases. It is worth pointing out that a few days prior, these numbers were smaller than what the Government Deputy of Mexico City reported, after applying 4,863 tests, in which 1,040 were confirmed cases. It is possible that these numbers could have grown due to the application of more tests.

Without a doubt, as a result of COVID-19 our attention has been focused on the critical situation in our prisons. However, it is worth asking ourselves: What are we willing to do to change it? Will we opt for viable alternatives such as Sanctions and Non-Custodial Penal Measures? Are we willing to boost measures that protect both human rights and penal procedures as alternatives to pretrial detention, without neglecting public safety? Will we eradicate the lag of penal execution procedures that could grant prerelease benefits?

Supervised Release: The Solution to a Pandemic Challenge

The COVID-19 pandemic has highlighted the needs and shed light on the deficiencies experienced by people living under custody inside penitentiary facilities, as well as confirming the shortcomings produced by a disproportionate and irrational use of prison. It is, without a doubt, the best time to redirect our attention to the strategy of the Release Supervision Authorities (Autoridades de Supervisión en Libertad). In face of the situation posed by the COVID-19 pandemic, the Units of Precautionary Measure (Pretrial Services Units), also known as UMECAS, due to its Spanish acronym, and Conditional Release authorities (Parole Services Authorities), which in some federal entities they belong to the same institution, have shared their experiences via videoconference. They have shown great promises as a solution, not just for depressurizing the penitentiary system, but as a shortcut to a short-term solution for improving the penal justice system and respect for human rights.

In 2011, an alternative was presented that would fundamentally solve the excessive use of imprisonment in Mexico. The State of Morelos created the first authority to implement supervision of precautionary release measures (Pretrial Services) for teenagers and a year later for adults. Its importance and relevance lied in the fact that, for the first time, we were able to witness a better option which favored people's freedom and human rights, without neglecting justice or resulting in impunity. This new element of the penal procedure has within its faculties the obligation to follow up on the 13 precautionary release measures in a timely manner. These measures can be applied before a judge decides to send a person to prison and without having received a conviction for a crime.

In the light of this scenario, we can observe that federal entities began creating authorities for the supervision of release measures (Pretrial Services), even before the issuing of the National Code of Penal Proceedings. Additionally, its publication has delivered an essential ingredient for the rationalization of the precautionary model, the so-called "evaluation of procedural risks." This evaluation gives authorities the ability to develop a technical opinion based on the principles of neutrality, objectivity, impartiality, and confidentiality that can be used by a judge to determine the ideal or necessary measures for each case. This implies that a person's criminal prosecution automatically should be imprisoned while waiting for a fair trial that would determine their innocence. The judge has the obligation to use the principle of minimum intervention according to each person's particular circumstances to determine the adequacy and proportionality of the measure and justify why it is the least harmful to the accused.

In light of these measures, we can assert that it is no longer about seeking a person's early punishment, but rather to ensure their presence during prosecution, guarantee the safety of the victim, the witness or the community, and avoid hindering the prosecution until it comes to determine an end of the culpability or innocence of the accused.

After the adoption of these measures the penitentiary system had a break from the extenuating pressure of its own context. For example, from January to September 2019, there were 28,619 people under supervision or 37% of the accused waiting to be prosecuted, while 34.1% (26,376 people) were given pretrial detention, and 12.9% (9,981 people) were allocated in prisons even in cases that were not classified as serious crimes under Article 19 of the Constitution. Additionally, statistics suggest that 16% of the accused (12,396) did not receive any kind of precautionary measures (SESNSP, 2019).

The Institute of Procedural Penal Justice (Instituto de Justicia Procesal Penal, 2019) conducted a study through its UMECAS (Pretrial Service Units) observatory in 2017, which revealed that on average, 78% of people given one or more precautionary measures complied with them. Furthermore, by 2018 the average rate of compliance for the country was 77% (SESNSP, 2018). Hence, it is relevant to acknowledge that the numbers were encouraging even before the expansion of the pretrial detention crime catalogue in 2019. However, it has been established that a 5-year evaluation is needed to assess efficacy in the use of release measures.

It is worth pointing out that alternatives to imprisonment do not constitute as improvisation; on the contrary, they are public policies that have been approved, evaluated and consolidated in other countries. An example of this is “Pretrial Services” in the United States, which have been operating for more than 50 years. These policies are promoted so that more of the states and counties’ justice systems opt out of pretrial detention and instead favor community supervised release measures.

In 2016, the National Criminal Enforcement Law also contemplated the creation of an authority for supervise conditional releases (Parole Services), with the intent of encouraging the use and monitoring of prerelease benefits and non-custodial sanctions such as, conditional, and early releases which people can gain before completing their sentence in its totality.

According to the National Monthly Penitentiary Statistic Notebook (Cuaderno Mensual de Estadística Penitenciaria Nacional), by May 2018 there were 38,148 people under supervised release, while in 2015 that number was as high as 42,519 people, contradicting the expectation set by this law since the number of people who have accessed a conditional release or a substitution to their custodial sentences has gone down.

Graph 3. *Supervised Released Versus Pretrial Detention* (2019)

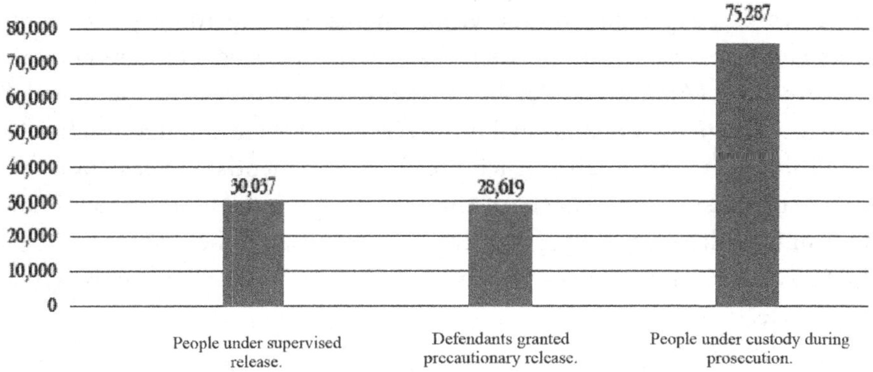

Source: Prepared by the author based on the December 2019 Cuaderno Mensual de Estadística Penitenciaria Nacional (National Monthly Penitentiary Statistic Notebook) and the September 2019 Modelo de Evaluación y Seguimiento de la Consolidación (Consolidation Assessment and Follow-up Model) by the SJP.

Overall, considering the number of people given pretrial measures and the number of parolees under supervision actively serving a sentence, the number reaches 66,767 people. This is the size of the challenge faced by supervised release authorities in the country, without considering that the overuse of pretrial detention and penitentiary overpopulation require the continuous bolstering of alternatives to imprisonment.

Final Thoughts

Due to COVID-19, we can discuss the actions taken by the Supervised Release Authorities. At first, just like other government entities, they were forced to adjust their activities, they opted for social distancing, and some units were closed to the public and others implemented sanitary protocols to continue providing attention as normal. Additionally, the use of technology plays an important role, as some units already have access to electronic GPS bracelets. Others decided to use phones and instant messaging apps like WhatsApp for monitoring. One thing is certain, the supervision does not stop, and in face of a pandemic the means that enable the activities of these authorities must be guaranteed.

It is worth pointing out that due to the encouragement of several parties, releases have been granted during the pandemic. In this sense, UMECAS (Pretrial Services Units) played an important role, by, in some cases, evaluating the people under custody that requested to have their pretrial detention switched to a precautionary release measure. At the same time, the cases of people under supervision increased. Regarding prereleases, estimated from March 31st to August 4th, 2020, 3,755 people were granted their freedom (Así Legal, 2020). For example, 660 people in the State of Mexico were granted conditional release, some of them through electronic monitoring (Jacinto, 2020), which meant an exponential increase of cases under supervision. The effects of the recently passed Amnesty Law (Ley de Amnistía) have yet to be seen. This law promised to be a way to add to the COVID-19 mass releases. However, to this day it has not been used in a single case.

In conclusion, it took worldwide public health concern for us to rethink the future of our prisons. The logical conclusion is that, on one side, we should stop deliberate admittances of "alleged offenders" into our penitentiary facilities, due to its economic and social cost. The question remains on how to do it, an alternative could be an objective case-by-case evaluation, opting for prison only on exceptional cases and instead pushing for supervised releases through UMECAS (Pretrial Services Units), thus, consolidating a public policy that could inspire reliance and trust in the public justice system.

Another approach suggests completing the "National Program for Penitentiary Depressurisation" (Programa Nacional de Despresurización Penitenciaria) advised by CNDH (2020). This is a coordinated effort between relevant penitentiary system authorities to promptly evaluate prerelease cases that fulfill the requirements stated by the law or belong to vulnerable groups in social reinsertion centers, considering that monitoring from the Supervision Authorities is vital to the person's social reinsertion. Medium and long-term measures should not be considered temporary programs resulting from the state of emergency; rather, these measures should be contemplated as an access to prerelease right that is ensured to everyone and that no one should be delayed from obtaining.

In this sense, the use of non-custodial sanctions established by the law, such as community work, may considerably favor a new reinsertion program. These programs should aim not solely punishing offenders, but to sensitize them on their social responsibility, thus, avoiding the adverse effects of unnecessary detention and redirecting state funds that are wasted in minor offence cases in prisons. Both strategies have the same objective: that prison becomes the exception and that it is used in a formal and rational manner, therefore, transforming prison into a space that is fit for social reinsertion and not for the undermining of human rights.

Bibliography

Acebes, J. M. (2020). Cómo evitar que las cárceles de América Latina se conviertan en una incubadora del coronavirus. The New York Times. Retrieved from: https://www.nytimes.com/es/2020/05/21/espanol/opinion/prisiones-covid.html

Así Legal. (2020). Mapa Penitenciario COVID-19. Retrieved from: https://asilegal.org.mx/mapa-penitenciario-covid-19/

Comisión Nacional de los Derechos Humanos. (2019). Diagnóstico Nacional de Supervisión Penitenciaria. Retrieved from: https://www.cndh.org.mx/sites/all/doc/sistemas/DNSP/DNSP_2019.pdf

Comisión Nacional de los Derechos Humanos. (2020). Informe especial sobre el estado que guardan las medidas adoptadas en centros penitenciarios para la atención de la emergencia sanitaria generada ante el virus SARS-CoV2 (COVID-19). Retrieved from: https://www.cndh.org.mx/sites/default/files/documentos/2020-07/IE_COVID19_Penitenciarios.pdf

Comisión Nacional de los Derechos Humanos. (2020). Pronunciamiento para la adopción de medidas emergentes complementarias en favor de las personas privadas de la libertad en la República Mexicana, frente a la pandemia por COVID-19. Retrieved from: https://www.cndh.org.mx/sites/default/files/documentos/2020-04/Pronunciamiento-personas-privadas-libertad-COVID19.pdf

Comisión Interamericana de Derechos Humanos. (2013). Informe sobre el uso de la prisión preventiva en las Américas. Retrieved from: http://www.oas.org/es/cidh/ppl/informes/pdfS/informe-pp-2013-es.pdf

Consejo Nacional de Población. (2020). Datos abiertos. Retrieved from: https://datos.gob.mx/busca/dataset/proyecciones-de-la-poblacion-de-mexico-y-de-las-entidades-federativas-2016-2050

Corte Interamericana de Derechos Humanos. (2020). Declaración 1/20. Retrieved from: http://www.corteidh.or.cr/tablas/alerta/comunicado/declaracion_1_20_ESP.pdf

Instituto Nacional de Estadística y Geografía. (2019). Censo Nacional de Gobierno, Seguridad Pública y Sistema Penitenciario Estatales. Retrieved from: https://www.inegi.org.mx/programas/cngspspe/2020/

Instituto de Justicia Procesal Penal. (2019). Observatorio UMECAs: En México, la mayoría de las personas con medidas cautelares en libertad las cumple. Retrieved from: http://ijpp.mx/acervo/noticias/item/1711-observatorio-umecas-en-mexico-la-mayoria-de-las-personas-con-medidas-cautelares-en-libertad-las-cumple

Jacinto, R. J. (2020). Suman 660 liberados de penales en Edomex por COVID-19. El Universal. Jacinto, R. J. (2020). Suman 660 liberados de penales en Edomex por COVID-19. El Universal. Retrieved from: https://www.eluniversal.com.mx/metropoli/edomex/suman-660-liberados-de-penales-en-edomex-por-covid-19

Novoa, M. (2020). Justice Reform puts Mexico at a dangerous crossroads.

Americas Quarterly. Retrieved from: https://www.americasquarterly.org/article/justice-reform-putsmexico-at-a-dangerous-crossroads/

Oficinas del Órgano Administrativo Desconcentrado Prevención y Readaptación Social. (2020). Cuaderno Mensual de Información Estadística Penitenciaria Nacional. Retrieved from: https://www.gob.mx/prevencionyreadaptacion/documentos/cuaderno-mensual-de-informacion-estadistica-penitenciaria-nacional

Organización Mundial de la Salud. (2020). Preparedness, prevention and control of COVID-19 in prisons and other places of detention. Retrieved from: https://www.euro.who.int/__data/assets/pdf_file/0019/434026/Preparedness-prevention-and-control-of-COVID-19-in-prisons.pdf

Penal Reform International. (2020). Global Prison Trends 2020. Retrieved from: https://cdn.penalreform.org/wp-content/uploads/2020/05/Global-Prison-Trends-2020-Penal-Reform-International-Second-Edition.pdf

Ramírez, S. G. (2019). Seguridad y justicia: plan nacional y reforma constitucional (primera ed.). Ciudad de México, México: Universidad Nacional Autónoma de México. SESNSP. (2018). Consolidación del SJP, Informe de acciones. Retrieved from: https://www.gob.mx/cms/uploads/attachment/file/416392/Capitulo_2._Etapa_de_Consolidaci_n_del_Sistema_de_Justicia_Penal.pdf

Secretariado Ejecutivo del Sistema Nacional de Seguridad Pública. (2019). Modelo de Evaluación y Seguimiento de la Consolidación del SJP. Retrieved from: https://sesnsp.net/mes/

The World Justice Project. (2020). Índice de Estado de Derecho. Washington DC. Retrieved from: https://worldjusticeproject.org/sites/default/files/documents/WJP-Global-ROLI-Spanish.pdf

Political Communication and the Pandemic

Maribel Flores

In Mexico, the health crisis caused by the pandemic has taken place in a political atmosphere marked by the distrust of institutions and political actors, a crisis in political representation, and governments' insufficient ability to handle it. These elements translate to a significant combination of democratic challenges in terms of legitimacy for decision making, governability, and the enhancement of a multilevel governance model. In sum, this is the consequence of public administration's deficient capacity for communication.

Challenges of Political Communication

Since Ancient Greece, politics have been studied as a human activity. Communication is inherent to the socialization process of the Zoon Politikon, or political animal, which is the only being capable of adapting to a political community, according to Aristoteles. However, Rus and Arenas (2013) point out that becoming this civic, political, or rhetorical animal, requires traits such as language to communicate or intelligence for project development qualities that allow establishing a form of coexistence in public society. Political decision-making and their implementation in communities are the results of communication—in the public sphere which implies the interaction with specific people and institutions producing a message exchange (Canel, 2010). Politics are communication, and in turn, communication is essential to politics; as the driving force behind the state apparatus, it upholds effective leadership and guides the community. Consequently, there are no politics without communication, as it is the medium and the means to a democratic government.

This process of dialogue and exchange between the government and its citizens meets specific functions in the political system on which democracy, governance, and governability depend. Canel (2010) emphasizes that communication is necessary at two different levels of politics: in the source of power and the exercise of power. To govern, communication should have a constant rhythm, given that it is important to consistently and systematically communicate political decisions due to the fact that it is impossible exert power without communication. In order for decisions to be transmitted and obeyed by society, they must be communicated. Among mass communication models, Laswell"s model published in the 1940s stands out; its functions focus on informing society about occurrences, then interpret them, and impacting public opinion. Thus, five elements to breach the gap between the government and its citizens in the process of communication were suggested. This would be done through a transmitter that would broadcast a message through a communication channel that would reach different receivers aiming to have an impact.

Currently, with the arrival of Information and Communications Technologies (ICT), it is imperative that political communication is strategic, given the use of devices that allow producing, storing, exchanging, and transmitting data between different information systems, enabling interpersonal interaction, collaboration, and multi-directionality. These tools play a substantial role in the production, exchange, dissemination, management, and access of knowledge; their accelerated innovation has influenced different scenarios, among which social relations, organizational structures, and public policies stand out (Cobo, 2009).

In the digital era, it is possible to access and contribute to information and the creation of ideas, allowing for bilateral exchange and interaction that favor development. In a democratic environment, political communication flows vertically (from the government to the citizens) and horizontally (among citizens). Although in the last few decades communication flow occurs in social media, the greatest challenge for politics and the form of implementing collective decisions is effectively broadcasting a message without clear centralization.

In this sense, public administration requires abilities for communication, as well as planning for communication when carrying public policies into effect. Now more than ever, governing implies communicating in a planned manner to make interaction with citizens effective and to create support during the decision-making process. Nevertheless, in the face of a crisis, the capacity to adapt to the environment's changes and to make adjustments to the governance plan is required. These changes and adjustments are extremely relevant during the turning point the pandemic represents, in which there is recognition of the emancipation of a citizenry that is more critical of public policies and willing to have an influence over them. Citizen monitoring and the evaluation of public policies will present a challenge to public administration and the exercise of political power. In this light, one must question whether governments are prepared to communicate effectively with the citizenry or if they will be prepared to answer to them. In this article, some of the main challenges regarding political communication in the context of the COVID-19 health crisis are laid out.

Timely Communication

In a context of uncertainty and complexity, it is essential to communicate precisely and promptly. Lack of information and transparency in public administration produces speculations and even fear among the population. This, in turn, promotes the spread of fake news, which hinders attention to the sanitary crisis, creating additional problems and greater social conflict. Silence translates to a power vacuum that affects governability and legitimacy when it comes to a lack of effectiveness in decision-making. Political communication is strategic since those who communicate politics do so to achieve a purpose or following a plan. It is persuasive and deliberate, especially during a crisis; it is designed to affect people's beliefs, attitudes, principles, or actions. Therefore, timely communication in these conditions is vital for continuity in governance.

Broadcasting a Valuable Message

Political messages are the guiding force of communication; they constitute a symbol of power that makes them significant in the public sphere. They are the content of what one intends to communicate and must be clear, empathic, and useful to the citizenry, especially during extraordinary circumstances. Political discourse enables, justifies, and transforms political action, seeking not only to represent a specific social reality but to convince, persuade, and re-signify as well. In public policies, different layers of an ideology through institutional logic, government practices, and citizen behavior are articulated. Discourse's practical function in power relations is assigning meaning through the process of ideologizing (Lamizet, 2002). Discourse pervades in the public policy cycle by directing public opinion through political language, which encompasses everything communicated in the political arena. Hence the importance of sending a valuable and meaningful message in the current situation. Given that, as Fabbri and Marcarino (2012) assert, political discourse is not only a place for information broadcasting, it is also one for its transformation.

Sharing High Quality Information Transparently

Information shared with citizens must be consistent, reliable, and communicated transparently. This responsibility must be taken on with honesty, sensibility, and attention to social concerns while listening, participating in dialogue, and incorporating any information from all sectors that might be useful to the public when handling the health crisis. This does not only require communication but coordination among different government spheres, the private sector, and civil society as well.

Transparency in governmental actions allows citizens to perceive a leadership style that shares reliable, consistent, and coordinated information. Nevertheless, throughout the pandemic, some leaders have turned to religion as a form of defense to face the health emergency, attempting to inspire trust and hope through discourse that refers to religious faith. In the midst of the pandemic, religious discourses have been introduced in Mexico. Some politicians have mentioned God in their messages to the population, even showcasing amulets that aim to grant personal protection to contagion and decrease society's concern. At the beginning of confinement, this was one of the methods used to reduce the pandemic's risk. However, reality surpassed the rhetorical strategies of those politicians who opted to discuss their religious faith. Crisis management is not handled by churches; rather, it is handled through the commitment of all citizens and their governments to reduce the risk of further contagion.

Therefore, turning to science to contain the virus and avoid making this pandemic one of the country's greatest tragedies is recommended. Greater social cohesion and civic awareness must be promoted—hence, the idea that politicians' message should transmit what health specialists seek to carry out. In the eyes of the public opinion, communication should happen coherently, guaranteeing to respect and abide by what is said through actions. People cannot be blamed for believing in an idea, but a leader will be evaluated by the public opinion when there is overwhelming evidence against it. The result of political communication will be approval or disapproval of political decisions made.

Strategically Handling Communication

A crucial figure when handling communication during this situation is the spokesperson, who makes information about the health crisis public in a proactive and transparent manner. The spokesperson or official representative must be an expert, a technician, whose function is to guarantee continuity in the information flow citizens must receive, in this case, regarding health specifically.

In governance, one must intervene strategically; press conferences, for example, usually aim to inspire trust and certainty in different government spheres. Press conferences are a tool for communication through which leaders define a position on topics to public opinion, solve crises, and solve questions about several topics related to governance plans (Estrada and Sanchez, 2019). A press conference's routine allows reporting back, but their use and frequency depend on each political leader. During the pandemic, the Mexican President, governors, and local authorities have carried out several conferences in diverse ways. At a federal level, there is the President's morning conference and another one in the evenings with health authorities. Additionally, local authorities conduct another one in which politicians and experts in the field converge.

Communications management requires public officials with expertise in the field, capable of laying down the government's agenda to the media, which will be questioning the country, state, or municipality's panorama as well as authorities' decision-making. Shared information should be standardized to avoid confusion, inconsistency, or wariness. Depending on the type of message that is being broadcast and on the type of audience being addressed, there should be a team of professionals in communication leading a strategic plan regarding the subject and capable of responding to a crisis. In current circumstances, there is no room for improvisation nor time to correct mistakes caused by inexperience or lack of skills that could have been prevented.

Counteracting Fake News

Communicating during situations of risk is a great challenge when governing since confusion and misinformation have been consistent during the pandemic. During the post-truth era, there is an overabundance of information that can spread massively and exponentially through social media, where going viral and political trends are prioritized through the sensationalism and dramatization of the news; this produces a greater political polarization in society.

Currently, rationality is separate from emotions in political decisions, and social upheaval has become the natural state of affairs; increasingly, contextualization, and relativization in the face of radical stances is fading. This is because as society becomes informed about public life matters, usually through social media, the fake news phenomenon grows and overwhelms journalism, which must interpret large amounts of information to tell the truth from different perspectives, as a consequence of the lack of reliable and verified resources necessary to complete its task.

In times of COVID-19, social media dynamics show that complexity evolves in real-time and requires the constant adaptation of decision-makers, such that government representatives' political outlook is not enough; dialogue, agreements, and negotiation are also required to implement public policies that solve public problems.

It has been long since communication stopped being another auxiliary department for public administration. Currently, implementing public policies essentially requires political communication to legitimize the government's decision-making and to establish interaction with society. Therefore, nowadays, it is vital to understand the context in which politics are carried out after social media and new technologies have made an impact, to recognize that they do not only alter the environment but practices and democratic political attitudes too.

Exercising Effective Political Leadership

Political leaders have handled the health crisis differently, few with greater success than others, but the vast majority have faced harsh criticism during the process of containing the pandemic. Across the three government levels, decision-makers are learning how to develop emergent leadership to manage their teams and citizenry. Political discourse is a key element when promoting cooperation among different working teams and sharing a message of trust and tranquility with society during moments of social turmoil without losing consistency between the speech and political behavior in order to avoid confusion, or rather, contradiction amongst the citizenry.

During a crisis, leaders are expected to reduce uncertainty and explain what happens, why it is happening, and what must be done. Dealing with crises has become a defining characteristic of contemporary governance, which requires leadership with the ability to adapt to the environment's condition.

Leadership style cannot be standard, as it depends on the individual's qualities and traits, but during a crisis, leadership is the driving force to produce organizational change and handle conflict. Implementing public policies is a political process that also requires technical rationality; therefore, leading this process requires responsiveness to reduce the existing gap between what is ideally conceived and what can be realistically done, especially in extraordinary circumstances (Pardo, Dussauge y Cejudo, 2018).

Decisions should be managed with political commitment, professionalism, rationality in decision-making, opportunity to act promptly, critical thinking, and modesty to recognize areas of opportunity. The government's functional structure is systematic when incorporating politicians' decisions and public officials' execution—recognizing that, although administrative posts are certainly not political, they have become politicized as a positive political attitude is required of them (Nieto, 2012).

During the pandemic, communities and members of organizations expect their leaders to reduce the crisis's impact while critics and political competition use social media to blame them and their policies. In this extreme situation, those in charge of creating policies must encourage collective learning from this experience, identifying political risks, and taking the opportunities they face, the traps they must avoid, and the paths they might pursue into consideration (Boin, 't Hart, Stern & Sundelius, 2005). Governments must take a step forward during the crisis with a plan for effective communication that can answer the most relevant questions proactively: What is truly happening? What are the biggest risks? What is the government doing? How are decisions being made? What do citizens need?

Although it is not possible to establish a direct correlation between an authoritarian political regime or a democratic one and the efficiency with which they handle the health crisis, world leaders' responsiveness has opened the possibility of inspiring trust (Fukuyama, 2020). The ability to produce public support toward organizations or the capacity to have social approval regarding political decisions is crucial in order for political leaders to carry out their jobs successfully and for citizens to perceive the possibility of a better future.

In this context, one must opt for an efficient communication strategy with the purpose of breaching the gap between what the government does, what public administration says it does, and what citizens perceive that is being done. Thus, avoiding the frustration of those who govern when they are unable to get their actions across, as well as that of those who are governed when they perceive their leaders' inefficiency, indifference, or inability regarding decision-making. Because of this, the effective communication of a decision for the public results in giving it added value. A good communication strategy is, in this sense, creating an intangible public asset (Canel, 2018).

Political legitimacy, or endorsing the system, is a priority dimension of public opinion, as reducing social support could entail political instability or a crisis. That is, a greater level of trust results in a greater margin to govern effectively, given that politicians possess the necessary legitimacy (Hetherington, 1998). In situations in which there is little trust, a government's poor performance and political scandals lead to a quicker deterioration and to governments' quicker loss of social support to lead (LAPOP, 2019). This is a worldwide phenomenon, but it has effects at a local level too; hence, that emerging political leaders must work in order to overcome political communication barriers in a democratic system: wariness, lack of credibility, and political polarization.

Although during the last few years society has become wary of politicians and the government in Mexico, support toward the democratic system has remained above 50% since 2004, reaching a turning point in 2016, in the six-year presidential term with the least social endorsement of the democratic system in over twenty years (Figure 1). However, there is a window of opportunity in 2020, according to the Latin American Public Opinion Project (LAPOP, 2019), support of democracy and Mexicans' satisfaction with the governmental system recovered in comparison to previous years.

According to the National Survey of Governmental Impact 2019 (Encuesta Nacional de Impacto Gubernamental, ENCIG), the perceived trust of political parties and of the government levels that they lead, such as institutions of political representation, increased during the past two years. On average, according to this measurement, the level of trust in institutions or social actors is as follows: federal government (51.2%), state government (40.5%), and municipal government (44.3%). This contrasts with Mexicans' level of confidence in their family members (86.8%) or public hospitals (63.3%).

In light of the situation and in the face of the previously described challenges, political leaders will have the opportunity of running political decisions legitimately through political leadership that can still rely on stable levels of trust during the health crisis. Finally, political leaders must develop communication skills to build trust and credibility by being consistent with their commitments to citizens while searching for the common good in an environment of political, economic, and social upheaval.

Graph 1. *Support of the Democratic System in Mexico 2004-2019*

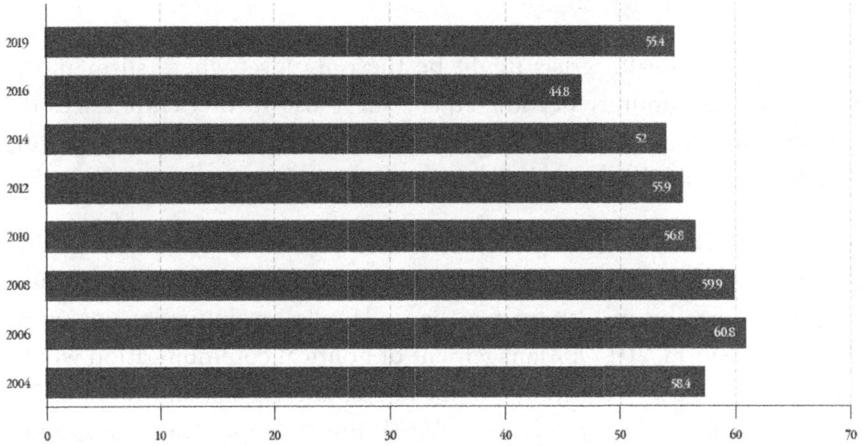

Source: Prepared by the author based LAPOP 2019 data

Graph 2. *Trust of Institutions in Mexico (2017-2019)*

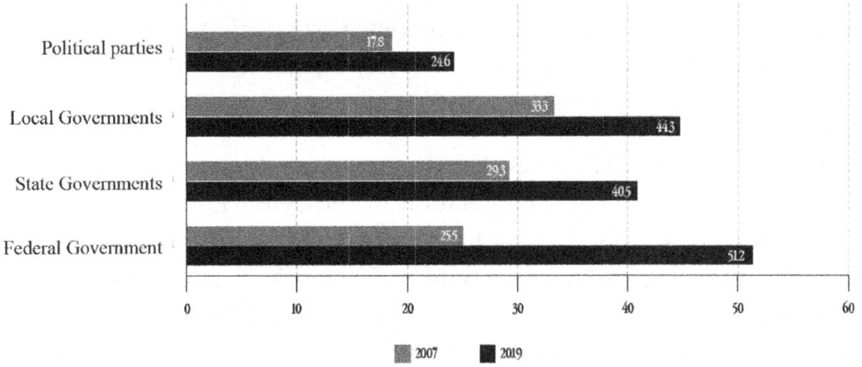

Source: Prepared by the author based on ENCIG 2019 data.

Recommendations

A pandemic is a phenomenon that completely alters public society, the space where human beings coexist, affecting every member of a community. Sadly, governance instruments are not designed to face all the implications that the pandemic entails; working on a recovery strategy to face the unfathomable consequences is necessary. Contemporary societies find themselves facing a phenomenon that demands transitioning into new forms of cooperative intelligence (Innerarity, 2020).

The COVID-19 health crisis might be the only level where all members of a political community become equal, but it also further emphasizes the economic and social inequalities prevailing in Mexico and globally, putting democratic consolidation to the test.

On a short-term basis, the government's functions should be focused on earning credibility, strengthening links, connecting emotionally, persuading, and mobilizing the institution for the collective resolution of upcoming challenges (Riorta, 2017). Management of political communication will be vital in the new community, one that can guarantee a shared responsibility for local political practices and global institutions. The institutional enhancement will depend on the government, the private sector, and civil society; boosting a good governance model will be a strategic wager for governments on a medium and long-term basis.

Leaders must communicate with honesty, empathy, and humanism, fostering a governance model; a relational or networking government, where openness to public-private interaction on a local-global axis is promoted. Leaders must allow (and conduct) different parties' participation in social action, prioritizing citizen participation, transparency, accountability, efficiency, and coherence (Nieto, 2012).

On a medium-term basis, a new beginning will imply deep changes in the way politics are done and the operation of the democratic system. Social interdependence will be decisive to the new reality that shall be recreated (Butler, 2020); the public arena should be "habitable" for everyone through the adapted interaction among social actors, in which social solidarity will be globalized by the new methods of coexistence in the digital era. Fukuyama (2020) has suggested a tri-dimensional formula that would be useful to face the crisis: starting with political leadership, society's solidarity, and the quality of institutions. Leadership will be charged with redefining the government's agenda, political entrepreneurship (collective decision-making), and building their reputation through political communication. Leadership is a solution to a series of problems which societies face when they attempt to reach common goals.

On a long-term basis, it will be necessary to start dynamic procedures for responsibility and learning, which are characterized by official investigations, blame management, public stunts, media scrutiny, and crisis exploitation (Boin, t' Hart, Stern & Sundelius, 2008). Overcoming the crisis should be understood from a holistic approach, recognizing that the challenges to be faced will not be limited to the emergency. The number of leaders that are currently unprepared to handle the crisis is not small, but what is most alarming is that post-crisis dynamics are ignored. In the future, through problem association, appropriate action plans should be chosen for the post-crisis phase in order to plan for the balance between failure and success. Leaders should be accountable for political decisions previous to the crisis while they learn to develop a post-crisis scheme to govern, which should be accompanied by a strategic communication plan.

To overcome the great communication challenges, discourse's role will be decisive to boost the new governance in management and coordination of society (Aguilar, 2018). The government will continue conducting the decision-making process, although in a new way that will require new institutions, a new relationship between the government and society, a government open to citizen participation, and a new public administration.

The networking government will be an alternative to way out of the crisis by expressing diversity and communicating collective decisions, hence the importance of political communication to establish social relations between independent parties that come together as a result of a public issues and are upheld and changed by interaction (Kooiman, 1993). Finally, governments should forge strong relations with parties involved in political communication, sharing true information about progress and achievements to face the crisis, and disseminating public policies that prepare the population for sustainable decision-making in a co-responsible and knowledgeable way.

Bibliography

Aguilar, L. (2016). *Democracia, gobernabilidad y gobernanza.* México: Instituto Nacional Electoral.

Boin, A., 't Hart, P., Stern, E., and Sundelius, B. (2005). *The Politics of Crisis Management: Public Leadership Under Pressure.* Cambridge University Press.

Butler, J. (2020). Sin miedo. *Formas de resistencia a la violencia de hoy.* México: Taurus.

Canel, M. (2010). *Comunicación política. Una guía para su estudio y práctica.* México: Tecnos.

———. (2018). *La comunicación de la administración pública. Para gobernar con la sociedad.* México: Fondo de Cultura Económica.

Cobo, C. (2009). El concepto de tecnologías de la información. Benchmarking sobre las definiciones de las TIC en la sociedad del conocimiento. Retrieved from: http://hdl.handle.net/10810/40999

Covarrubias, O. (2012). Diez retos de la administración pública en clave de coordinación. Retreived from: https://www.redalyc.org/articulo.oa?id=676/67624803002

Estrada, L., and Sánchez, D. (2019). "La comunicación política de los líderes neopopulistas americanos" en *Foreign Affairs Latinoamérica* 19 (4), 72-78. Retrieved from: http://revistafal.com/numeros-anteriores/fal-19-4/

Fabbri, P., and Marcarino A. (2002). El discurso político. Retrieved from: http://www.designisfels.net/revista/la-comunicacion-politica-transformaciones-del-espacio-publico

Fukuyama, F. (15 April 2020). The crisis of trust. Retrieved from: https://www.ft.com/content/a42-ba47c-2433-410f-8c5d-1753d4728570

Fundación IDEA. (2017). Resiliencia urbana en América Latina. Una guía breve para autoridades locales. Retrieved from: http://www.fundacionidea.org.mx/posts/49

Hetherington, M. (1998). The political relevance of political trust. *American*

Political Science Review, 92 (4), 791-808.

Instituto Nacional de Estadística y Geografía. (2019). Encuesta Nacional de Calidad e Impacto Gubernamental 2019. Retrieved from: https://www.inegi.org.mx/programas/encig/2019/

Innerarity, D. (2020). *Pandemocracia. Una filosofía de la crisis del Coronavirus,* Galaxia Gutemberg.

Kooiman, J. (1993). *Modern Governance: New Government-Society Interactions*, Sage.

Lamizet, B. (2002). Semiótica de lo político. Retrieved from: http://www.designisfels.net/revista/la-comunicacion-politica-transformaciones-del-espacio-publico

Latin American Public Opinion Project. (2019). Cultura política de la democracia en México y en las Américas, 2018/19: Tomándole el pulso a la democracia. Retrieved from: https://www.vanderbilt.edu/lapop/mexico.php

Levitsky, S. and Ziblatt, D. (2018). *How Democracies Die.* New York: Crown.

Nieto, A. (2012). *El desgobierno de lo público.* Barcelona: Ariel.

Open Government Partnership. (2020). Guía de Gobierno Abierto y Coronavirus: Respuesta abierta + Recuperación abierta. Retrieved from: https://www.opengovpartnership.org/wp-content/uploads/2020/07/Gui%CC%81a-de-Gobierno-Abierto-y-Coronavirus.pdf

Pardo, M., Dussague, M., and Cejudo, G. (2018). *Implementación de políticas públicas. Una antología.* México: CIDE.

Sapienza, S., Iyer, N., and Veenstra, A. (2015). Reading Lasswell's model of communication backward: Three scholarly misconceptions. Mass Communication and Society, 18(5), 599-622. Retrieved from: https://www.tandfonline.com/doi/abs/10.1080/15205436.2015.1063666?journalCode=hmcs20

Shepsle, K. (2016). *Analizar la política: Comportamiento, Instituciones y Racionalidad.* México: CIDE.

Creative Economy and Knowledge Economy

Esteban Santamaría

Innovation and Creativity: The Tools to Overcome the Pandemic

When this article comes to light, the effects of the pandemic will surely continue. Some of those effects have already been identified. For instance, The International Labor Organization (ILO) indicated that a large number of people will move into the informal sector as a result of the crisis, and that seven out of ten small business might not survive.

Despite the list of negative effects of the pandemic, three elements will help the world move forward: 1) Innovation, which can be seen both, in medicines and in the tools created to solve new problems and needs, such as ventilators for the critically ill; 2) Creativity, noticeable every time people watch a movie on digital platforms; and 3) Ingenuity, present in the current pursuit of new solutions with increasingly limited resources.

Therefore, creativity, innovation, and ingenuity could be the strategic factors that may contribute to face some of the problems caused by COVID-19. The suggested elements are summarized in two proposals: the knowledge economy and the creative economy. Both have been present in Mexico for many years, with achievements and mistakes as any other model. However, their potential impact shows that they are viable options to support economic growth, at the national and local level, as long as they are correctly implemented and address the institutional challenges that have been identified as limitations of their success (Benavente & Grazzi, 2017).

To face the pandemic effects on the alternatives proposed here, relevant stakeholders in society must be able to act accordingly. The government must make institutional, legislative, and public policy changes; the private sector must seek new ways to produce and commercialize its products and services; society must be willing to adapt and consume the products and services under new schemes. In that way, the chances to get ahead of the crisis will be greater.

According to Mangabeira (2005), moments of crisis are suitable to generate thoughtful and necessary changes to implement a knowledge economy. The real challenge is to take advantage of this opportunity to make the changes that allow the country to become prosperous and innovative from a long-term perspective. Those States that develop superficial measures, without having a diagnosis and a well-defined objective, will be the most affected regardless of the measures taken. On the contrary, it is possible that some negative impacts may be accentuated such as inequality and the digital gap.

Understanding Knowledge Economy

The knowledge economy is the accumulation of capital, technology, technology-relevant capabilities, and science in the conduct of productive. Through this, it is possible to increase the income and wealth of a population, while reducing social backwardness. Therefore, the United Nations Agenda 2030 underlined Science, Technology, and Innovation (STI) as the key tools for achieving The Sustainable Development Goals (SDG).

The theoretical perspective on this economy gained strength more than two decades ago. Primarily driven by the World Bank, and especially since the first study on the knowledge-based economy of the Organization for Economic Co-operation and Development (OECD), which recognized the benefits of public policies focused on promoting STI and creativity in some countries (1996). According to Powell and Snellman (2004), there are at least three interpretations of knowledge economy as an economic theory, which assumes that investing in knowledge will generate social and economic change.

Figure 1. *Interpretations of Knowledge Economy*

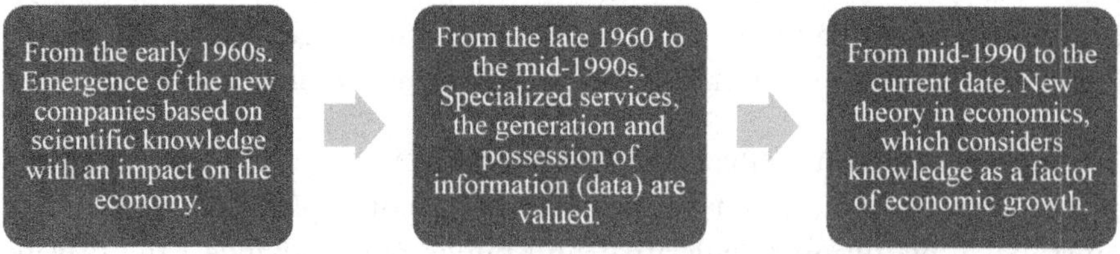

Source: Prepared by the author based on Powel and Snellman, 2004.

The aforementioned evolution is due to the investment made by people in their education and professionalization. Not only to get a better job (first two blocks), but now even more than before, it is key to be more competitive, or as a requirement to keep a job (last block). The impact of constant investment in the generation of new knowledge is usually reflected in the products and services offered in the market, increasing, or decreasing their value due to their presence or absence.

Nevertheless, the success of this economy is conditioned to the generation of changes in legislation, institutions, and public policies in at least four areas: education, culture, politics, and innovation. If this is not done, there is a possibility that it will not work; and this limitation would not be attributable to the model, but to its improper implementation.

The effect of these reforms would lead to changes in matters such as the collaborative culture by improving trust and cooperation between individuals, crucial both for generating innovations and for implementing them. However, as stated by Villareal et al. (2016), within the skills to innovate that are most sought after and least found in Mexico, teamwork is in first place and honesty in fourth place, which shows the lack of cooperation and trust among Mexican society.

If the changes and good dissemination are implemented appropriately, as stated by Mangabeira (2005), the knowledge economy would have the following effects in Mexico:

1. Generation of inclusive economic growth.
2. Reduction of the economic inequality caused in established market regimes, through progressive taxation followed by the redistribution of the social spending.
3. More advanced products with the potential of changing human life and with the capacity to generate a transcendental change in the economic activity.

Finally, a study by Gaona et al. (2017), which measured Mexico's knowledge economy and compared it with six other countries including the U.S., South Korea, Brazil, among others, showed that its impact is just above Argentina. Despite of the evidence of the benefits on economic growth in certain countries of investing more in the knowledge economy, in Mexico, the evidence shows that the impact of this practice has been incipient.

Understanding Creative Economy

According to Benavente and Grazzi (2017), creative economy is a group of activities in which ideas are turned into cultural goods and services, whose value is or could be protected by the Intellectual Property Rights (IPR). As stated by the same authors, creative economy is mainly constituted by three elements:

1. Recognition of creativity, art, and culture as productive initiatives.
2. The relationship with the generation and utilization of the IPR, especially the author's rights (copyrights).
3. The direct role in these activities in the value chain that transform ideas into products.

Creative economy, still quoting Benavente and & Grazzi, is made up of three main concepts: Traditional and artistic activities; creative industry, and the activities that bring creative support to traditional industries. This can be seen more clearly in Figure 2.

Figure 2. *Areas and Elements That Constitute the Creative Economy*

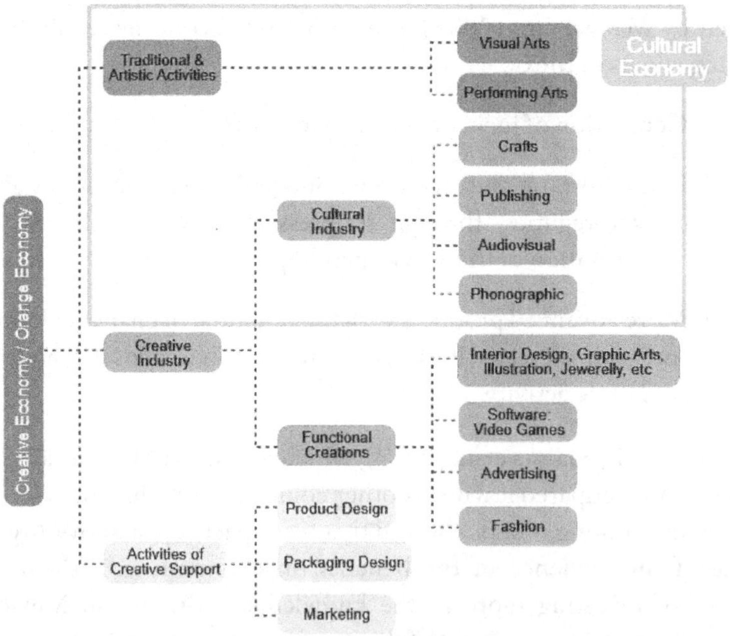

Source: Prepared by the author based on Public Policies for creativity and innovation: promoting the orange economy in Latin America and the Caribbean, Benavente & Grazzi, BID, 2017.

The relevance of the creative economy is internationally recognized, so much so that the United Nations Conference on Trade and Development (UNCTAD) has a specific program on the subject. As proof according to UNCTAD (2019), it contributes 3% of the world's Gross Domestic Product (GPD).

An example is Nigeria, where Nigerian cinema or Nollywood, is the yearly the second-largest producer of films, additionally, it is responsible of the generation of one million jobs, which positions it as the second source of job after agriculture, favorably impacting its GDP (Santamaria and Flores, 2018).

Just as in the knowledge economy, in the creative economy, it is also necessary to address at least three aspects for its dissemination (educational-cognitive, socio-moral, and legal-institutional). If applied correctly, it is expected to have at least the following benefits.

1. Generation of jobs, especially those related to the cultural and creative sector.
2. Support for economic growth, potentially with a social impact.
3. Promotion of a country's patrimony and culture, having an impact on the productive sector such as tourism, exports, or Information and Communication Technologies (ICT).

Nowadays, there are very few studies that allow identifying the creative economy impact in Mexico. However, a study conducted by the World Intellectual Property Organization (WIPO), identified that the economic impact of industries based on creativity is the most important; to mention an example, between 1998 and 2003, the creative economy contributed 4.77% of the GDP at the national level (Marquez-Mees, Ruiz Funes and Yaber, 2006).

From Crisis to Opportunity: The Implementation of the Knowledge Economy and the Creative Economy

A country that took positive advantage of a crisis was South Korea. Between 1997 and 1998, the government made a turnaround, generating profound institutional, legal, and public policy changes. Until this moment, those commonly known as Chaebol (large companies that were the engine of the economy and concentrated a large part of the productive activity) had been key in the development and growth of that country for decades; however,

Figure 3. *Chaebol and Economic Development Until 1997*

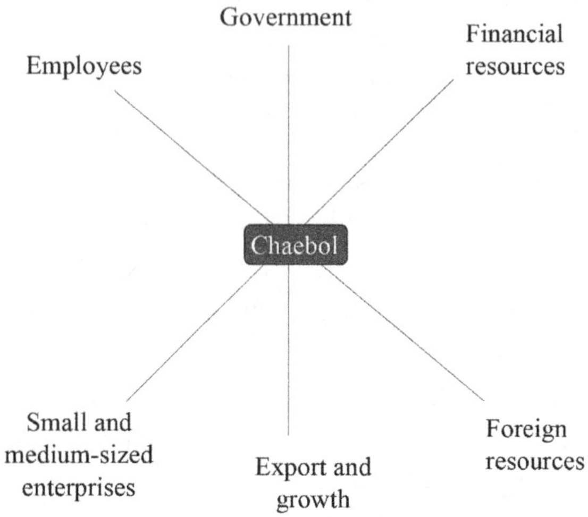

Source: Prepared by the author based on Phil-Sang Lee, Economic Crisis and Chaebol Reform in Korea.

they were also considered as one of the culprits of the crisis, due to the domino effect they caused (Lee, 2000).

Figure 3 illustrates how South Korea's performance allowed it to grow at 8 percent annually for many years, but it was also the "Achilles heel" that led to the crisis in 1997—a centralized system in which the investment base was mainly focused on the Chaebols, for them to be the principal engine of exports and the growth of the country, but at the same time increased the economic imbalance because of the enormous dependence on a few companies.

The government quickly reacted with various measures, for example, institutionalizing in the same year of the crisis, the Inter-ministerial Council for Informatization Strategy that was directly led by the President of Korea, and that had to implement and develop a cross informatization policy of the whole country through collaborations among different ministries (Ure, 2008). Two years later, in 1999, the Ciber Korea 21 initiative was implemented, bringing with it laws, funding, new institutions, and programs focused on strengthening the ICTs in the country.

Currently, South Korea occupies one of the top positions in the main innovation indexes or rankings. As an example, the impact of its investment in the creative industries was recognized in 2019 when the movie *Parasite* won the Academy Award from the Academy of Motion Picture Arts and Science of the United States. Another effect of its investment in ICT and the actions mentioned in the previous paragraph lay in the fact that the country became one of the pioneers in sectors such as online gaming. Korea's leadership in these matters may seem quite distant for Mexico, but it should be remembered that only fifty years ago that country was far behind in almost everything, compared to Mexico (GPD, education, exports, etc.).

From then on, the country continued with institutional, legislative, and public policy changes to implement its version of the creative economy. It has even become a state policy, as the President stated in her inauguration speech that "A creative economy, designated as the country's new growth strategy will generate new jobs and markets through the convergence of science and technology with information and communication technologies. Based on Korea's imaginativeness, creativity, business, and culture this strategy will provide long-term growth for Korea" (Geun Hye, 2013).

This example serves as a reference, except for the obvious differences of the current context. A central fact is that manufacturing was at the core of the Korean economy at the time of its crisis. The entry of the new United States–Mexico–Canada Agreement (USMCA) will indeed be a great help to overcome the pandemic effects; however, the protectionist measures that are been taken in several countries with which Mexico has a business, especially with the United States, force the government to look for alternatives that complement this free trade agreement.

Example of the Performance of the Knowledge Economy and the Creative Economy in Times of Crisis

The creative economy has shown more resilience to worldwide economic crisis than traditional manufacturing industries (UN, 2010). For example, during the 2008 financial crisis, while the world trade was contracting by 12% after a drop in demand, trade in goods and services grew at a rate of 14% annually from 2002 to 2008, reaching US $594 billion (El País, 2011).

Despite the serious distortions in internal offer and demand, and that most of the economic sectors have been affected including trade and the finances generated by the pandemic (World Bank, 2020), the technological segment dedicated to entertainment has been exempted. As an example, the shares of

Netflix are reaching new historical highs as the demand for its products and services continues to rise significantly (FINECT, 2020).

Regarding the knowledge-based economy according to the OECD, while the 2008 economic crisis affected the STI of all the countries, it also pushed a new path towards a "new productive revolution, fostered by science and technology" (2016). The reason was that some countries identified that through STI they could improve their production and at the same time become more competitive, which would have an effect on the companies, helping them to get out of their predicament.

Likewise, another study of the OECD (2012) also identified that the 2008 crisis demonstrated the weakness of some sectors, such as the automotive industry. This allowed countries like South Korea and China to test the effects of their work and investment in STI during previous years, which helped them to face the situation in a better light, besides, it was key for the positioning of large companies focused on innovation.

In summary, both economic proposals have proven to be effective in times of crisis. The evidence shows that their success was due to taking timely, correct, and cross measures. The countries that failed to do so, missed the opportunity to bring a profound change, and suffered some consequences as the inequality gap increased.

Conditions for the Implementation of the Knowledge Economy and the Creative Economy

The success of the implementation of both proposals depends on an integral work, starting from a diagnosis, the intervention of experts and an evaluation phase. Furthermore, as already mentioned, it is necessary to address at least three fronts simultaneously and address with accuracy about what must be done on each one: educational-cognitive, socio-moral, and legal-institutional. Doing so represents a profound change in the short-term, but with the most significant benefits in the long-term.

Currently, there are some experts that question the viability of these models, even Mangabeira (2019), one of the principal promoters of the knowledge economy expressed that from his perspective the effects have proven to be modest. The reason: the inappropriate design and implementation of the necessary policies. He considers that knowledge, innovation, and profits are still concentrated in a few companies. Moreover, he expressed that the efforts of numerous countries to change the situation have been scarce. The result is therefore not surprising.

Figure 4. *Steps to Implement Changes*

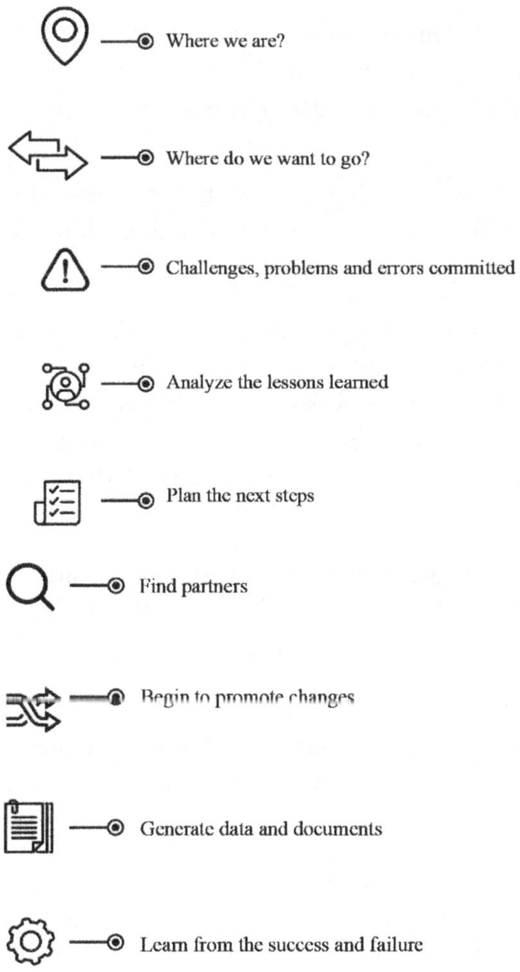

Source: Prepared by the author based on "Intellectual Property, Creativity and Innovation for the Development of Mexico: Ideas and Proposals from the Civil Society," Santamaría and Becerra, Caiinno, 2017.

In other words, the problem is not in these economic models, but rather in their design and implementation; this premise also applies to any other model that pretends to be used to overcome the effects of the pandemic. First of all, it is necessary to understand each of these proposed models, what they are, what they offer, and what is needed to implement them. If we do not start from there, according to the evidence, the effects will be limited and could generate negatives externalities that could have been foreseen and avoided.

In order to implement these models, it is suggested to follow the steps presented in Figure 4, which are a pathway to enhance the chances of success (Santamaría and Becerra, 2017) and see them as a cycle that should be repeated:

1. Where we are? It is suggested to make a broad diagnosis at the beginning to have a perspective that allows identifying all possible opportunities and problems.

2. Where do we want to go? Based on the results the priorities and the directions to follow can be determined, considering that human and economic resources will probably be insufficient at the beginning. Ideally, given the emergency, it is recommended to focus on the sectors where there are strengths or those that can generate more impact.

3. Challenges, problems, and errors committed. It is ideal to identify the challenges and the failures of the strategies, both our own and those of other governments.

4. Analyze the lessons learned. The information obtained should be useful to identify what was done well and not so well; likewise, it is ideal to generate new information used as a reference for the decision making.

5. Plan the next steps. Certainly, it is urgent to address all the sectors of the economic proposals, and although they must be addressed transversally, it is important to plan where, when, and how to act.

6. Find partners. Direct and constant collaboration with stakeholders is key. Their contribution will help to identify needs and opportunities, as well as support the implementation of the actions.

7. Begin to promote changes. With clarity about what must be done,

it is possible to start promoting and implementing the necessary changes. It is also important to design a strategy to convince all the stakeholders of their feasibility.

8. Generate data and documents. It is essential to document the information on actions taken and their results. This practice should be systematized and will be useful for future decisions.

9. Learn from the success and failure. It is necessary to carry out an evaluation in order to identify what does and does not work and the areas of improvement. Omitting this would be a serious mistake.

The aforementioned steps are a suggestion, and they will depend on the type of sector prioritized, so for example, supporting innovation through an increase in the number of invention patents requires different ad hoc measures than supporting the audiovisual sector.

Finally, it is also ideal for governments to leverage new technologies such as big data and artificial intelligence for the implementation of the new economies proposed. In the literature, a certain homogeneity can be found regarding the government and public administration in their approach with artificial intelligence: the efficiency is upgraded with the use and implementation of new technologies such as artificial intelligence and big data. Obviously when they are properly designed, supplied with data, and well used.

Examples of Actions in Response to the Pandemic: Cases in Spain and Brazil

On March 6, Spain launched several measures to support the cultural sector and taxation in order to deal with the pandemic (Government of Spain, 2020). These measures include actions to support companies through schemes that facilitate financing and cash flow in various sectors. Moreover, these actions considered support for workers, especially those vulnerable due to the pandemic situation. The decree is based on a brief and concrete diagnosis, followed by a very precise definition of the objectives, scopes, and actions.

These actions contemplate support schemes by sectors, since each one has unique characteristics that require a differentiated approach. Among the sectors considered are included the scenic arts and music, cinematography and audiovisual arts, books and contemporary art, and others.

Another example is Brazil. According to Santos-Duisenber (2020) the country implemented some of the following measures: 1) Law for the Cultural Emergency, which contains a variety of actions such as three months economic support to people working in the creative sector, as well as tax exemptions for up to six months; 2) At the subnational level, states like Rio de Janeiro and Brasilia also implemented financing and support schemes for the industries in the sector; and 3) Online events such as "Lives Solidarias" raised millions of dollars to battle COVID-19.

Table 1. *Science and Technology Policy Responses to the Pandemic in LAC*

Category	Measures implemented	AR	BR	CL	CO	CR	HN	MX	PY	PE	UY
Support for scientific research projects	Calls for Covid-19 oriented research	x	x		x		x	x	x	x	
	Strategic research projects finance										x
Support for innovative scientific-technological projects	Calls for pandemic related innovation projects	x	x	x	x			x		x	x
	Hackathons									x	
Institutional measures	Scientific advice for decision making								x	x	
	Inter-institutional coordination of scientific and technological actors			x		x		x			
	Organization of university-led research initiatives to the pandemic		x			x		x			

Source: Prepared by the author based on "Responses to COVID-19 from science innovation and productive development," Inter-American Development Bank, 2020.

In regard to the knowledge economy, some countries have taken different measures with different approaches to support the STI. Some of these actions included fostering research initiatives to face the COVID-19 impact, and to improve the competitiveness. Meanwhile, the IDB (2020) recently published a study with some of the STI policy interventions that are being implemented by some of the Latin American and Caribbean (LAC) countries as a response to the crisis.

Looking to the Future: The Economics of Ingenuity

The knowledge economy and the creative economy are very effective alternatives to face the crisis we are facing. Their benefits have already been described, as well as the general conditions for success. But it is also true that the present and the future require new measures because, in addition to the changes generated by the pandemic, other phenomena such as automatization or artificial intelligence will arrive faster and possibly with more force. Besides, other problems must be considered, for instance, the effects of climate change, among others. For that reason, it is necessary to begin to start proposing a new model that consolidates the best of these economic proposals, but which also includes a new perspective.

That option may be ingenuity. Not all is uncertain, the change that the world economy will undergo in the short-term, regardless of the pandemic, has already been analyzed by several authors, higher education institutions, and international organizations. The role that people play is going to change in many aspects, especially in the labor field. Hence, it is suggested to consider a model in which humans' skills and qualities become key to face the challenges ahead. Ingenuity therefore will be of great help, especially with the purpose to collaborate with new technologies and artificial intelligence.

Bibliography

Banco Interamericano de Desarrollo. (2020). *Respuestas al COVID-19 desde la ciencia, la innovación y el desarrollo productivo*. Washington, D.C.: Banco Interamericano de Desarrollo.

Banco Mundial. (2020). La COVID-19 (coronavirus) hunde a la economía mundial en la peor recesión desde la Segunda Guerra Mundial.

Retrieved from: https://www.bancomundial.org/es/-news/press-release/2020/06/08/covid-19-to-plunge-global-economy-intoworstrecession-since-world-war-ii

Benavente, J. M., and Grazzi, M. (2017). *Public policies for creativity and innovation: Promoting the Orange Economy in Latin America and the Caribbean*. Washington, D.C.: Banco Interamericano de Desarrollo.

Conferencia de las Naciones Unidas sobre Comercio y Desarrollo. (2019). How the creative economy can help power development. Retrieved from: https://unctad.org/news/how-creative-economy-can-help-power-development

Dos Santos-Duisenberg, E. (2020). Brazilian culture and creativity during COVID-19: Solidarity and lives. Retrieved from: https://pec.ac.uk/blog/brazilian-culture-and-creativity-during-covid-19-solidari ty-and-lives

El País. (2011). Economía creativa: una apuesta creíble. Retrieved from: https://elpais.com/diario/2011/07/10/negocio/13103036 71_850215.html

FINECT. (2020). Amazon y Netflix: 2 gigantes que desafían la crisis del coro navirus. Retrieved from: https://www.finect.com/grupos/Investing com/articulos/amazon-netflix-2-gigantes-desafian-crisis-coronavirus

Gaona Rivera, E., Sierra Castill, J. M., and González Gómez, D. X. (2017). Economía del conocimiento: El caso de México en comparación con seis países. *CIMEXUS* 13 (2), 65-82.

Geun Hye, P. (2013). A new era of hope. Retrieved from: https://www.newsd.admin.ch/newsd/message/attachments/33379.pdf

Gobierno de España. (2020). Real Decreto-ley 17/2020, de 5 de mayo, por el que se aprueban medidas de apoyo al sector cultural y de carácter tributario para hacer frente al impacto económico y social del COVID-2019. Retrieved from: https://www.boe.es/diario_boe/txt.php?id=BOE-A-2020-4832

International Labour Organization. (2020). COVID-19 crisis and the informal economy: Immediate responses and policy challenges. Retrieved from: https://www.ilo.org/wcmsp5/groups/public/---ed_

protect/---protrav/---travail/documents/briefingnote/wcms_743623.pdf

Lee, P. S. (2000). Economic Crisis and Chaebol Reform in Korea. Retrieved from: https://www8.gsb.columbia.edu/apec/sites/apec/files/files/discussion/PSLee.PDF

Mangabeira Unger, R. (2005). *The Knowledge Economy*. Paris: OCDE.

Mangabeira Unger, R. (2019). Rethinking the knowledge economy. *American Affairs Journal*, III(2), 3-24.

Márquez-Mees, V., Ruiz Funes, M., and Yaber, B. (2006). The Economic Contribution of Copyright-Based Industries in Mexico. Retrieved from: http://www.wipo.int/export/sites/www/copyright/en/performance/pdf/econ_contribution_cr_mx.pdf

Naciones Unidas. (2010). Informe sobre la economía creativa. Retrieved from: https://unctad.org/es/Docs/ditctab20103_sp.pdf

Naciones Unidas. (2020). Guidebook for the Preparation of Science, Technology, and Innovation (STI) for SDGs Roadmaps. Retrieved from: https://sustainabledevelopment.un.org/content/documents/26001Guidebook_STI_for_SDG_Roadmaps_First_Edition_clean0323.pdf

Organización para la Cooperación y el Desarrollo Económicos. (2012). OECD Science, Technology and Industry Outlook 2012. Retrieved from: https://www.oecd.org/sti/sti-outlook-2012-chapter-1-innovation-in-the-crisis-and-beyond.pdf

Organización para la Cooperación y el Desarrollo Económicos. (2016). Perspectivas de la OCDE en ciencia, tecnología e innovación en América Latina 2016. Retrieved from: https://www.oecd-ilibrary.org/docserver/9789264303546-es.pdf?expires=1593703358&id=id&accname=guest&checksum=28228219AFBBFA4AD447EF34D283D14A

Powell, W., and Snellman, K. (2004). The Knowledge Economy. *Annual Reviews*, 30, 199-2020.

Ramírez, C. M. (s/f). *La Economía del Conocimiento en México: Condiciones para el Crecimiento Económico*. México: UNAM.

Santamaría, E., and Becerra, D. (2017). *Propiedad intelectual, creatividad e innovación para el desarrollo de México. Ideas y propuestas desde la sociedad civil.* México: Centro de Análisis para la Investigación en Innovación, A.C.

Santamaría, E., and Flores, H. (2018). El país africano que llegó a producir más películas que Hollywood. Retrieved from: https://elpais.com/elpais/2018/03/02/planeta_futuro/1520008043_445523.html

Villarreal Peralta, E. M., Santamaría Hernández, E., Díaz Gómez, E., Ballesteros Páez, M., Birtwistle, S., Rodríguez Hernández-Vela, C. E., and Urueta Rico, W. (2016). Habilidades para la innovación. Retrieved from: https://www.britishcouncil.org.mx/sites/default/files/resumen_ejecutivo_habilidades_para_la_innovacion.pdf

Civic Education in Times of the Pandemic COVID-19: A Reflection Towards the Challenges in Mexico

Cecilia García

Citizenship and Pandemic

The word "citizenship" has been a term regularly and repeatedly used over the last few years in Mexico. Once the political parties became aware of the deterioration they were experiencing, and the apathy they were provoking among the electorate, they began to use the concept of citizenship in order to "refresh" the political system in Mexico, and thus, the entire party structure. Nevertheless, the term is not limited to political or electoral matters. On the contrary, citizenship must play a relevant role in the daily life of any person.

Sadly, Mexico is not a country defined by its active citizen participation. According to the National Survey of Political and Citizen Practices (Encuesta Nacional de Cultura Política y Prácticas Ciudadanas ENCUP), published in 2012, only 1 out of 4 citizens in Mexico can find a common interest with another citizen regarding the resolution of a public problem. In contrast, the same survey shows that three-quarters of the population is very proud to be Mexican. In a nutshell, it is easier for Mexicans to participate in events related to the Mexican National Soccer team or during certain holidays like Day of the Dead, which embraces national identity, than when they must participate in public affairs.

The citizen's behavior during the pandemic has been a significant factor in the transmission and spread of the virus. According to official information, the first confirmed case of COVID-19 in Mexico occurred on February 27th. Almost a month later, the federal government implemented a national social distancing program and declared a quarantine that involved the closure of schools, businesses, mass events, and meetings in order to slow down the probability of contagion. Since then, it started a political, social, and economic crisis whose consequences in the medium and long term have not been fully estimated. A year later from the beginning of the pandemic, Mexico has not properly complied with the official measures to mitigate the spread of the virus.

International agencies such as the United Nations Economic Commission for Latin America and the Caribbean (UN-ECLAC) have emphasized that the crisis resulting from COVID-19 could cause a setback of more than two decades in terms of development, not only because of the increase in poverty and marginalization, but also because of the lack of growth and opportunities for the region and its inhabitants. Unlike other crisis, the current one is not limited to the financial and economic spheres; instead, it is a health crisis that is also impacting the social and political spheres worldwide.

The Pandemic in a Convulsive Political Context

The pandemic occurred at a very particular time for the world. Before the pandemic, global political systems were already undergoing structural changes that impacted their credibility among citizens. Democracy was facing great challenges such as the weakening of institutions, citizen apathy, the emergence of populist currents, etc. The 2019 Democracy Index developed by the Intelligence Unit of the British magazine *The Economist* stood at 5.44, which represented a decrease of 0.04 points compared to 2018. It represented the worst result since the study was first conducted in 2006.

Globally, 2019 is remembered as a year with a broad presence of citizen protests in the streets, instability in governments democratically elected, freedom violations, power abuses, among others. Latin America, the most unequal region in the world and with a large part of the systems currently in the process of consolidation, represented a fertile ground for the growth of social discontent generating political instability in countries such as Argentina, Bolivia, Brazil, Chile, Guatemala, and Venezuela.

According to the analysis conducted by IDEA International (2020) in its Global State of Democracy Index, Mexico has not had an optimal management to reduce the costs derived from the pandemic. One of the elements pointed out by the analysis was the concern about the constant confrontation and criticism of President Andres Manuel López Obrador with media, private actors, and political opposition about its strategies to face the pandemic.

The Covid-19 pandemic has intensified a difficult scenario regarding the respect of rules, as well as the lack of trust towards the government and its institutions from its citizens. In fact, the pandemic could strengthen authoritarian attitudes and values leading to the detriment of the democratic values in the world.

Citizenship: An Often Repeated But Little Understood Term

There are countless definitions of the meaning of citizenship. Following the purpose of this policy brief, it is considered appropriate to use the definition proposed by T. Marshall (1950) in his essay on "Citizenship and Social Class." He states that citizenship is a status granted to the members of a community, divided as follow:

- Civil dimension: those rights related to physical freedom. Freedom of speech, thought, religion, the right to hold property titles, equality within the law, such as the right to a natural and a formal process, freedom of association and opinion, among others. In the context of the COVID-19 pandemic, these rights have been limited due to the need of States to impose confinements to reduce the infection rates, which opened a new window on how to exercise these rights during a pandemic.

- Social dimension: the dimension where Marshall locates rights such as the right to education, security and access to health services. In the context of the COVID-19 crisis, it has been demonstrated that, although it is the State's responsibility to safeguard social rights, different stakeholders (private, social, academic actors) must share responsibilities for maintaining them.

- Political dimension: it concerns the rights related to voting and the political organization. In Mexico, citizenship is acquired at 18 years of age. At that moment, it is possible to obtain an ID card from the National Electoral Institute (Instituto Nacional Electoral) for voter registry, in which the right to vote can and must be exercised, every time elections are called.

In this regard, in the framework of the analysis of citizenship, one of the most recurrent debates is to understand the existing position between rights and obligations: Which came first? Rights or Obligation? A large number of citizens always put rights first. In the same manner, it is common to hear that the State must guarantee rights—which is true—but it is also questioned: What about obligations? Likewise, considering the current context of the pandemic, it is imperative to ask ourselves: What about the responsibilities that citizens must fulfill to guarantee a rule-bound environment and an optimal and peaceful interaction with others?

The debate should not be positioned in the prioritization of rights over obligations or vice versa. On the contrary, the analysis should focus on the permanent search for a balance between the interactions and the relationships in society. The concept of citizenship should be understood as the set of values, knowledge, and attitudes that allow people to get involved in public affairs with responsibility. In this way, the rule of law becomes a condition that emerges among the members of a society and the State.

As in war economies, in a crisis such as the COVID-19 pandemic, the role of the State becomes essential and central. Nevertheless, citizens' actions are equally important. Therefore, it is also imperative to ask ourselves: What to do when the citizens do not abide by the rules or do not respect the rule of law? What are the costs for the countries, including Mexico, and their societies? An effective alternative to stop the spread and the effects derived from COVID-19 is through strict compliance of confinements by adopting the public health measures established by the authorities.

The situation we are living in should motivate us to reflect about citizens' role in the reduction of contagion; thinking about whether our decisions are respectful towards other members of society. This might be the only way to confront this crisis of public health and to ease the economic effects on multiple sectors at the international level. In other words, as long as citizens abide by the rules properly, the faster this crisis will be over, and the economic effects may be less than estimated.

However, in the last months of 2020, while the number of COVID-19 cases increased in Mexico, confinement and sanitary measures were less respected by a large part of Mexican society. It is evident that millions of citizens in Mexico have not respected the rules during confinement in the context of the pandemic. People continue to gather in enclosed places, do not wear properly their masks, or do not wear them at all. This series of behaviors can be explained due to the deterioration of the rule of law, weak trust in institutions and authorities, and a lack of civic and democratic values.

The "Mexico: Country Report" published in 2015 by INE and El Colegio de Mexico (COLMEX) developed an interesting analysis about the quality of the citizenship and the trust in institutions. According to this report, 37% of participants agreed that there was limited respect for the law in Mexico, and 29% said there was no respect for the law at all. The total of both numbers (66%) speaks of a majority with a misperception of the functioning of the rule of law; not to mention conscious impunity that undermines the culture of legality.

Graph 1. *How Much Do You Think That Laws Are or Are Not Respected in Mexico?*

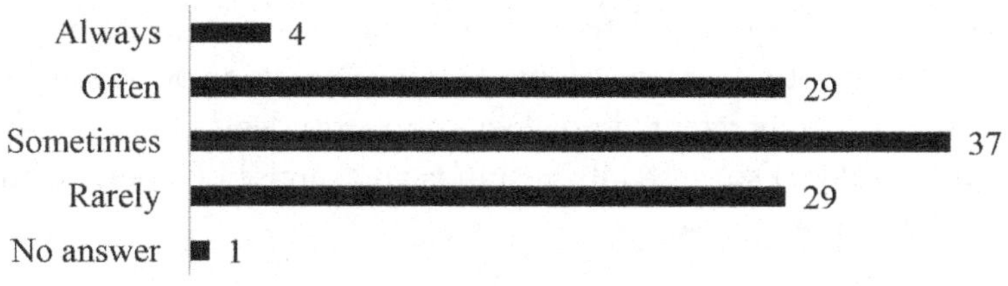

Source: Prepared by the author based on INE and Colmex, 2015.

On the other hand, this same analysis refers to the low level of trust existing within the Mexican population towards its institutions and authorities. As shown in Graph 2, with values under 35%, deputies, political parties, labor unions, police officers, and judges are the least trusted figures at the national level. In summary, this situation puts Mexico in a complex moment to effectively address the health emergency. Without trust and compliance with the rules by citizens, it is and will be difficult to mitigate the pandemic in the country.

Graph 2. *Level of Trust in Institutions, Political and Social Organizations*

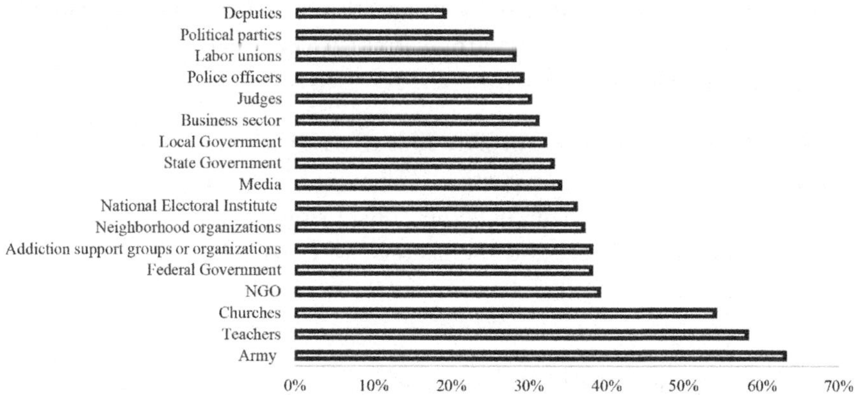

Source: Prepared by the author based on INE and Colmex, 2015.

What Can Be Done in Order to Change This Situation? Political Culture, Civic Education, and Social Capital

In 1983, Almond and Verba conducted a comparative study about the attitude and opinion of the political system in five countries. Based on this analysis, they defined civic culture as the set of knowledge, evaluations, and attitudes that a certain population has towards several aspects of political activity and its political system. However, when speaking of citizenship, the concept does not only refer to knowledge and attitudes, but rather; as Naval and Laspalas (2000) suggest, citizenship is an exercise of a permanent and purely social nature.

Political culture goes far beyond the rules of social interaction, that allow the harmonious relationship between the individuals that constitute society. Political culture establishes a clear distinction between what is considered socially acceptable and what is not; it consists of educating individuals to behave in accordance with the norms and to be able to relate to each other in a socially determined environment of reciprocity and respect.

In synchrony with the political culture, civic education must be reinforced, which is understood as the development of values, attitudes, and knowledge of the inhabitants of a country; this according to their political culture from the interpersonal, intrapersonal, and cognitive spheres. Civic education shall not be static, instead, it must address the current needs of society. In this sense, civic education needs to cover at least the following areas: a) the analysis of the ethical principles of social interaction; b) the recognition of the various forms of human groupings and the different ways of organizing collective life; and c) initiation in the various ways of participating in social and political life (Ibañez, 1998).

Another of the central aspects of civic education is that it must be approached from an interdisciplinary perspective (Naval and Laspalas, 2000), in which different areas of knowledge converge, thus, bringing together visions that explain relations in society and the exercise of citizenship. This means that citizenship development shall be immersed in everyday living, and not only in politics.

In the living context of COVID-19, it is increasingly relevant to talk about these two concepts: to understand that we live in a society and that we affect others with the decisions we make as individuals. For example: to wear or not to wear masks, to respect or not to respect the safe distance measures, to open or not to open a business that is not indispensable, to gather or not to gather with family or friends, have positive or negative implications on others.

How to achieve a harmonious relationship between the individuals that constitute a society? One alternative can be strengthening social capital. As Putnam (2000) states, social capital is considered as an enabler to a more efficient and cohesive society, because, when people organize themselves either to solve common problems or to demand more from the authorities, they build societies with larger development. Besides, Putnam defines social capital as a virtuous circle of interaction, reciprocity, and trust.

Figure 1. *The Virtuous Circle of Social Capital*

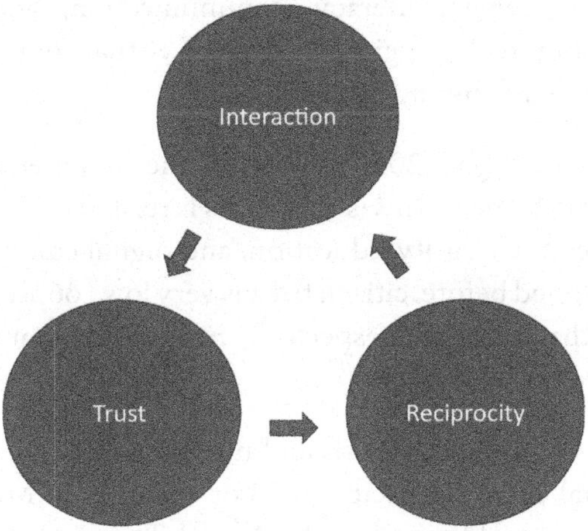

Source: Putnam, 2000.

This means that increasing the relationship between people in a country's community, allowing them to interact and establish common objectives will generate greater trust in the medium and long term. A clear example about this last assumption is underlined in the "Mexico: Country Report" (2015), which estimates that 38% of the people surveyed mentioned that a friend from their neighborhood (community level) is their most important contact, which coincides with the premise that cohesion networks at the communitarian level are the most relevant and abundant. Therefore, another important challenge for Mexico is to build social capital for everyone, regardless the socioeconomic level, education, political or religious ideology, race, or gender. Simply, more social capital leads to a better society.

What Can Be Done in Order to Reinforce Civic Education in Mexico?

(1) Reinforcing Civic Education in a Digital Context

Although the social distancing and confinement measures imposed by governments around the world have helped to reduce considerably the wave of COVID-19 infections; these measures have also initiated a debate over their impact on the exercise of the freedoms and rights of the population. In other words, isolation, or confinement to reduce the spread of the virus should not impede citizens to organize and participate in public decisions.

Along with this pandemic, people have started to talk about digital citizenship, which requires the development of basic competencies such as: promoting and strengthening digital literacy, communication, and collaboration through information technologies, creation of virtual content, security, and resolution of problems, among others.

For Martinez and Vega (2020), one of the requirements of citizen participation in digital platforms is trust. This is related to the transformation of processes based on security, education, and digital culture. In the case of Mexico, as mentioned before, citizen trust is very low (66% of the population do not believe that rules are respected), making the transition to digital citizenship much more complex.

On the other hand, connectivity should not be ignored as a nodal element to promote digital citizen participation. For example, in Mexico, according to the INEGI's National Survey on the Availability and Use of Information Technologies 2019 (Encuesta Nacional sobre Disponibilidad y Uso de Tecnologías de la Información en los Hogares, ENDUITH), there are 20.1 million households with Internet access, which represents 56.4% of the total. This demonstrates, without a doubt, a large digital gap. Although the use of cellphones is growing —86.5 million, according to the same survey mentioned above—not all people use the Internet for the same purposes. According to reports from Hootsuite and We are Social (2020), in Mexico, people use more than 60% of the Internet to navigate on social networks.

In this order of ideas, building trust and constant training are fundamental elements towards the reinforcement of digital citizenship in Mexico. For these reasons, the following strategies are proposed:

- Reinforcing civic education in the school curriculum during the confinement. Currently, civic education cannot be learned traditionally. It is suggested to use innovative mechanisms in the teaching-learning process and to use virtual resources such as YouTube. Generating attractive content should be one of the main interests of the Ministry of Public Education (SEP), aimed at improving the lack of strengthening social skills of girls and boys who are not attending schools.

- It is imperative that the civic education promoted by SEP counts with the competencies that children need to achieve digital citizenship in the coming years.

(2) Civic Education as a Cross-Cutting Component in the Development Programs

Nowadays, more than ever, the way how citizens behave is fundamental for the development and prosperity of the countries. For this reason, civic education should be the cross-cutting component of public policy in the coming years. It is not about valuing civic education as an isolated element; instead, it should be conceived as a fundamental piece in the construction of better societies.

This can only happen with actions and strategies that are sustainable and consistent over time:

- Civic education as a cross-cutting component in national, state, and municipal development plans. Including civic education in everyday life will bring about an increase in social capital and trust in the institutions, as well as respect for laws ad norms.

- To date, the Federal Expenditure Budget (Presupuesto de Egresos de la Federación, PEF) has no specific budget programmed for civic education. Although different entities have this competence (SEGOB, INE, INAI, SEP), none of them has a specific budget reserved for this area. Thus, a public policy without a budget becomes a good intention, nothing more. In this sense, it is proposed that SEP, jointly with INE and INAI, lead a civic education program with a specific budget at the national level.

The challenges currently faced by humanity because of the pandemic are only "the tip of the iceberg." In the next decades, dealing with public health, food, and environmental problems derived from human irresponsibility will be more common than ever.

Citizenship education should be a priority from the government, corporate, social, and academic spheres. Civic education is not an accessory or an electoral platform, but rather influences daily activity and healthy interaction in societies that are increasingly pluralistic and complex.

Finally, more empathetic citizens, capable of recognizing their value in the public space, aware of the importance of following the rules, and above all, understanding that people cannot live in isolation, will constitute a watershed for the development of better societies and individuals in the future, in Mexico and worldwide.

Bibliography

Comisión Econónica para América Latina. (2020). Coyuntura, escenarios y proyecciones hacia 2030 ante la presente crisis de COVID-19. Observatorio COVID-19 en Ameríca Latina y el Caribe. Retrieved from: https://www.cepal.org/sites/default/files/presentation/files/coyuntura_escenarios_2030_crisis_covid-19_ab.pdf

European Union. (2020). The Digital Competence Framework 2.0. Retrieved from: https://ec.europa.eu/jrc/en/digcomp/digital-competence-framework

Ibáñez-Martín, J. (1988). Formación cívica y sistema democrático. *Revista Española de Pedagogía,* 46(181), 441-451.

Instituto Nacional Electoral y El Colegio de México. (2015). *Informe país sobre la calidad de la ciudadanía en México*. México: INE.

International Institute for Democracy and Electoral Assistance. (2020). The Global State of Democracy Index. Retrieved from: https://www.idea.int/gsod-indices//#/indices/countries-regions-profile?rsc=%5B70%5D&covid19=1

Marshall, T. (1950). *Ciudadanía y clase social.* Cambridge: University Press.

Martínez Mancilla, Y., and Vega, M. (2020). *Gobernanza participativa de la inteligencia artificial*. Washington D.C.: Banco Interamericano de Desarrollo.

Naval, C. y Laspalas, J. (2000). *La educación cívica hoy. Una aproximación interdisciplinar*. Pamplona: Eunsa.

Putnam, R. (2000). *Bowling Alone: The Collapse and Revival of American Community*. New York: Simon & Schuster.

The Economist. Democracy Index. (2019). Retrieved from: http://www.eiu.com/Handlers/WhitepaperHandler.ashx?fi=Democracy-Index-2019.pdf&mode=wp&campaignid=democracyindex2019

Verba, S. and Almond, G. (1963). *The Civic Culture: Political Attitudes and Democracy in Five Nations*. Princeton University Press.

Profiles

Carol Daniela Aceval Carmona

Carol is currently working as the General Director of Execution of Penalties, Security Measures, Supervision of Precautionary Measures, and Conditional Suspension in the State of Durango (Probation and Pretrial Services), where she promotes networks for social reintegration, restorative justice, and collaborative work with local and national authorities, business owners, and nonprofit organizations. She holds a Bachelor's degree in Law and a Master's degree in Law with a mayor in Constitutional and Administrative Law from Juárez University of the State of Durango (Universidad Juárez del Estado de Durango), as well as a Master's degree in Public Administration by the Sonoran Institute of Public Administration (Instituto Sonorense de Administración Pública). Moreover, she earned distinguished certifications such as the Program on Justice Innovation in the United States by the Justice Studies Center of the Americas and the Center for Court Innovation. Carol is a co-author of the book *Las medidas cautelares: el tope a la puerta giratoria* edited by Tirant Lo Blanch and the National Institute of Criminal Sciences (Instituto Nacional de Ciencias Penales).

Juan Carlos Baker Pineda

Mr. Baker is a professor at the Panamerican University (Universidad Panamericana) in Mexico City, where he teaches undergraduate and master's degree courses on international trade, international finance, economics & international affairs. Previously, he developed a twenty-year career in the Mexican federal government, in areas such as international trade negotiations and foreign affairs, culminating as Vice Minister for Foreign Trade between 2016 and 2018. As Vice Minister, he was responsible for designing, coordinating, and implementing Mexico's trade policy in North America, Europe, Asia, and Latin America. Mr. Baker led Mexico's team in the negotiations for the modernization of the United States–Mexico–Canada Agreement (USMCA, formerly NAFTA), the Free Trade Agreement between Mexico and the European Union (FTA EU-MX), and the Comprehensive and Progressive Agreement for Trans-Pacific Partnership (CPTPP), among others. After his service in the federal government, Juan Carlos founded the firm Consultores Internacionales Ansley, which offers a wide range of services aimed at helping leaders and decision-makers in the public, private and social sectors to achieve their objectives.

José Carlos Espinoza Lanz

Mr. Espinoza is the Director of Operations in Kybernus, a social program that supports the development of leaders based on values that strengthen the capacity of society to improve their surroundings, in coordination with public, private, and social stakeholders for the creation of social value in Mexico. During his tenure, he has been involved in the design and implementation of social leadership training programs, as well as mentoring and monitoring local initiatives in the 32 Mexican states. He was the Director of "*Haz Futuro,*" an educational initiative aimed to align and articulate Higher Education Institutions knowledge supply with the needs of the industry. Moreover, José Carlos has served as Educational Advisor of CONAFE, CONALEP, and Plantel Azteca, executing diagnosis reports, evaluations, strategic planning, and curriculum development projects. As a specialist in peace education, he has collaborated with nonprofit organizations and designed leadership and peace culture workshops focusing on conflict resolution. He holds a Bachelor's degree in Philosophy and a Master's degree in Education.

Maribel Flores Sánchez

Maribel is the Division Director of the School of Social Sciences and Government of the Monterrey Institute of Technology (Tecnológico de Monterrey) in Puebla. As a Full-Time Professor of the Political Science and International Relations Department, she develops national and international projects on educational innovation and academic programs in democracy, political communication, and public entrepreneurship. She is a member of the Transparency and Anticorruption Initiative of the School of Government and Public Transformation. Moreover, as a specialist in management and public policy with more than 20 years of experience in public, private and social sectors in Mexico, the United States, and Spain, she develops citizen participation and anti-corruption strategies for strengthening civic culture. She has a master's degree in Public Management from the Complutense University of Madrid (Universidad Complutense de Madrid) and certifications in International Relations, International Cooperation and Integration in Latin America, Sustainability and Project Evaluation.

Cecilia García Montoya

Cecilia is the co-founder and General Director of Despierta, Cuestiona y Actúa, A.C. For more than ten years, she has been designing, implementing, and evaluating programs focused on children and young people around civic education and political and social participation as a strategy to increase citizen competencies and social capital. She worked at the National Institute of Transparency, Access to Information and Protection of Personal Data (Instituto Nacional de Transparencia, Acceso a la Información y Protección de Datos Personales) and in the Presidency of the Republic. Cecilia has been an adviser for local governments on issues related to childhood and youth in Mexico. Finally, she has a master's degree in Political Communication and Strategic Governance from The George Washington University (GWU).

Rosangel Hernández Mendoza

She is Director of Research and Analysis in Consultores Internacionales Ansley and Coordinator of the Editorial Committee of Trade Tank MX. She has worked in the Office of the Presidency of Mexico, the Ministry of Environment and Natural Resources, and the Ministry of Economy, specializing in elaborating and analyzing strategic reports, particularly in policy and international trade. She earned a degree in International Relations at the Autonomous University of Nuevo León (Universidad Autónoma de Nuevo León) and a master's degree in Asian and African Studies, specializing in China in El Colegio de México.

Pedro Manuel Lichtle Fragoso

Mr. Lichtle is a consultant on innovation policy in Mexico. He is a lecturer at the Monterrey Institute of Technology (Tecnológico de Monterrey). Pedro specializes in innovation, tourism, and public policy, and he has extensive professional experience in the federal government of Mexico. He has also collaborated with local governments, academic institutions, and international organizations. He has a M.S. in Public Policy and Management from Carnegie Mellon University and a B.S. in Economics from the Center for Economic Research and Teaching (Centro de Investigación y Docencia Económicas) in Mexico.

Marcela Reynoso Jurado

Marcela is currently working as Operational Division Head, in the National Evaluation and Operation Unit, of the Mexican Institute of Social Security (Instituto Mexicano del Seguro Social), where she performs analysis, design, and evaluation of public policies. During the pandemic, Marcela collaborated with the Oxford Coronavirus Government Response Tracker, a project that systematizes public policy actions to face the COVID-19 pandemic. She previously served as a legislative advisor at the Federal Congress, where she analyzed and ghostwrote initiatives regarding Gender Equality, Transparency, and Public Security. She holds a master's degree in Public Policy from the University of Oxford and a master's degree in Gender and Law from the National Autonomous University of Mexico (Universidad Nacional Autónoma de México).

Esteban Santamaría Hernández

Esteban Santamaria is one of the founders and Director of the Mexican think tank CAIINNO (Centro de Análisis para la Investigación en Investigación). He has carried out research and projects that have served as a reference for elaborating state development plans, initiatives of law, among other activities for governments, private sector, academia, and international organizations. He worked at the Inter-American Development Bank (IADB) as a specialist consultant in intellectual property, innovation, and creative economy, leading projects, and publications in those fields. Mr. Santamaría has represented Mexico and Latin America in activities organized by institutions such as the United Nations Conference on Trade and Development, the World Intellectual Property Organization, the United States Patent and Trademark Office, among others. He earned his Law Degree and Master's in Law & Economics from the Autonomous University of Puebla (Benemérita Universidad Autónoma de Puebla), where he graduated *Cum Laude,* and the LLM in Intellectual Property Law by The George Washington University (GWU), awarded with the Fulbright scholarship. Currently, he is pursuing a doctorate in politics and government.

Daniel Tapia Quintana

Daniel Tapia is the founder and Executive Director of Genera, a public policy consulting firm specializing in public policy, program evaluation, advocacy, and forecasting analysis. During his tenure, Mr. Tapia has developed several projects with international and local clients, including the LEGO Foundation, the W. K. Kellogg Foundation, The World Bank, the Inter-American Development Bank (IADB), RAND, Instituto Natura, Technopolis, The Global Fund for Children, The British Council, USAID, Vía Educación Grupo Salinas, Ministry of Economy, Ministry of Interior, Ministry of Infrastructure, among others. He is the author of national and international articles and publications such as a report for UNICEF – East Europe and three book chapters on such diverse subjects as education, youth, informal economy, poverty reduction, and public policy. In 2015, Mr. Tapia was selected to participate in the Aspen Institute Fellows' first generation in Mexico. Additionally, he is a member of the Technical Committee of the chapter FUNED – Puebla and is a Mentor of young participants in the Banamex Excellence Program. Mr. Tapia holds a Master's degree in Education in International Education Policy from Harvard University and a Bachelor's degree in International Relations from Universidad de las Americas Puebla.

Made in the USA
Monee, IL
30 March 2024

55479322R00075